SUPERSIZED FOR CHALLENGED EYES

Super Large Print Variety Puzzles

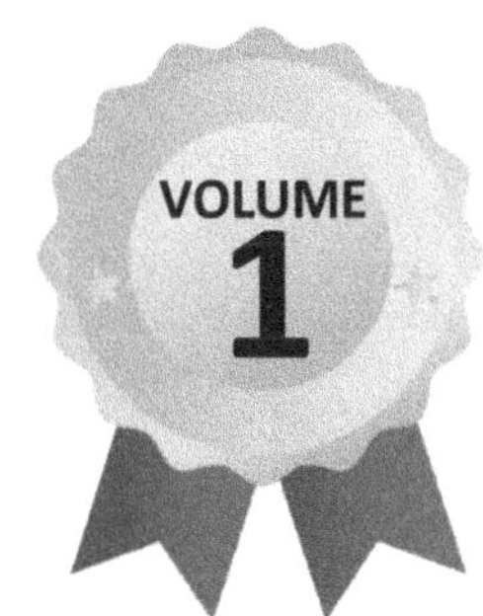

48 Fun Challenging Puzzles

WORD SEARCH
SUDOKU
NUMBER SEARCH
WORDOKU

Easy to See - Easy to Handle

All Scripture verses quoted herein are taken from the English Standard Version (ESV) of the Bible.

Copyright © 2019 Nina Porter

All rights reserved. This book or parts thereof may not be reproduced in any form, stored in any retrieval system, or transmitted in any form by any means – electronic, mechanical, photocopy, or otherwise – without prior written permission of the publisher, except as provided by United States of America copyright law.

**SUPERSIZED FOR
CHALLENGED EYES
PUZZLE BOOKS**

are dedicated to my mom

Helen Louise Foster Clark
1917 - 2016

Mom loved word search puzzles, and when she could no longer see the "large print" versions, I began to create puzzles for her that she could see in a format that was easy for her arthritic hands to handle. As her eyesight grew worse, the print became larger, and – they became *supersized!*

May this book be a blessing to you!

~ Nina Porter

Welcome to Supersized for Challenged Eyes. You'll find that these puzzle books are easy to read and fun to solve.

We hope you'll enjoy the variety of puzzles and enjoy many hours of puzzle solving fun.

Find all the Supersized Books at amazon.com/author/ninaporter

Sign up to receive a Free Printable Word Search Puzzle each week and download a Puzzle 4-Pack at

SupersizedPuzzles.com

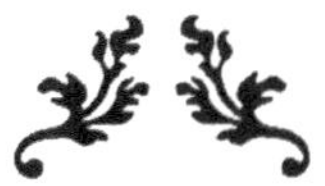

Word Search
Puzzle Section

Enjoy the following fun themed puzzles, with Bonus Words to find, Scripture verses, and Quotes.

Words can be forward, backward, up, down or diagonal, and may overlap.

ALL CREATURES GREAT & SMALL

```
E N Y E L S E L I D O C O R C
X L O W R E K V G J K M H P F
O S A A U M M I P N R X P E M
S A E H Y R R U U T W F T L A
T B L S W A A M R O D E D E R
R S J L F N P B K H R N R P M
I N H F I I Z C B E I R S H O
C B E A H R E L K I B N Y A S
H I R C R G O R F C T I O N E
R P U X H K H G E S U O M T T
```

BEARS	GECKO	OSTRICH
BIRD	GIRAFFE	RABBIT
CHIPMUNK	GORILLA	RHINO
CROCODILE	LEMUR	SHARK
ELEPHANT	MARMOSET	SHREW
FROG	MOUSE	WHALE

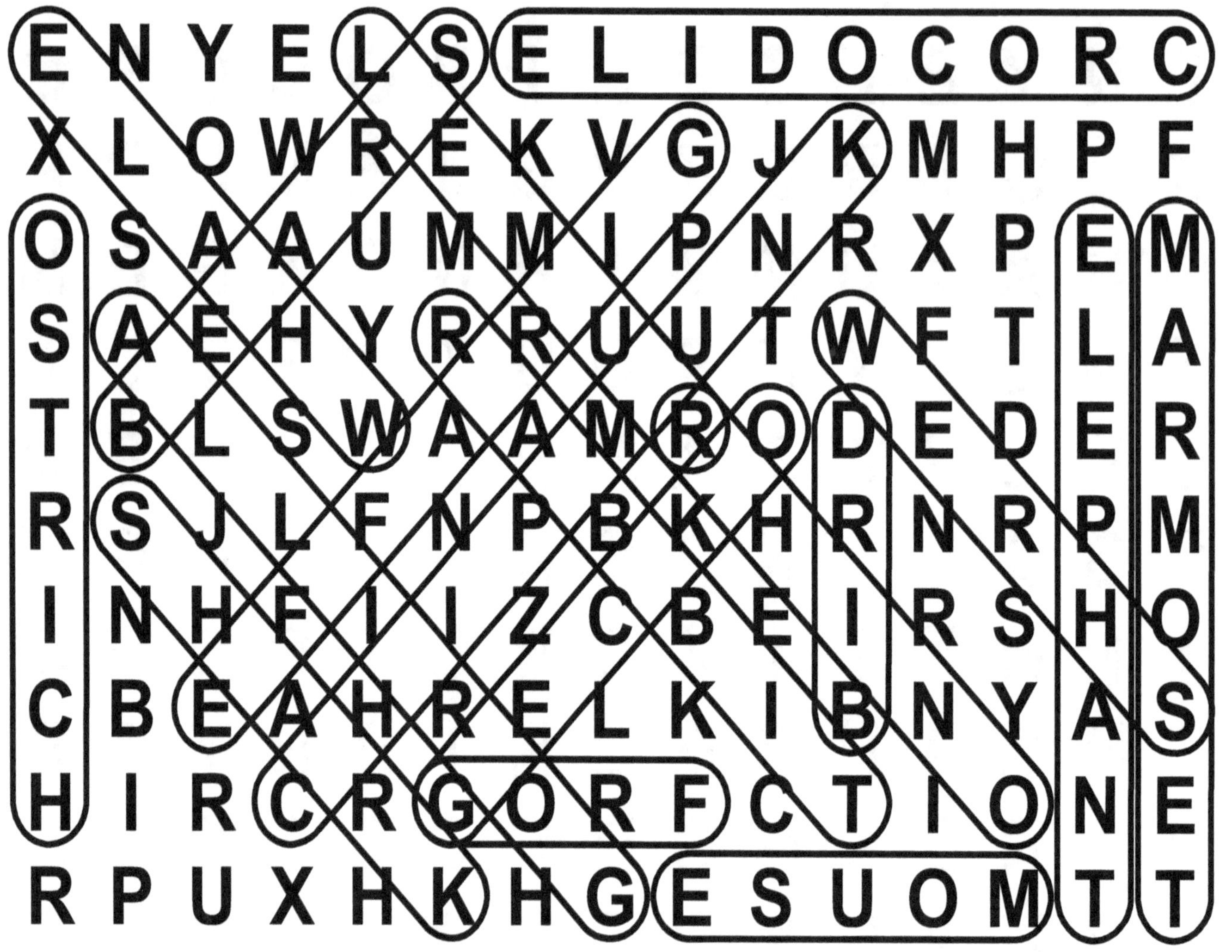

> "All creatures great and small, all things wise and wonderful: the Lord God made them all."

> ~ Cecil F. Alexander,
> Hymns for Little Children, 1848

BY THE NUMBERS

```
C R V T P I E C E R Z K S C R
S H T S J L T Z S C E R A D N
G O E N T N O D L G C B V B O
N Y J C U O N R S O N A I G I
I M P O K E C R E I A N N N T
N T C R D I E K N F R K G I A
R C A I I T N V S Y U I S L N
A N V X U C E G C L S N G L O
E I K R E S E L A S N G D I D
D E N I T S I N V O I C E B G
```

ACCOUNT	EARNINGS	REFUND
BANKING	INSURANCE	RETURN
BILLING	INVEST	SALES
CHECKING	INVOICE	SAVINGS
DIVIDENDS	PRICE	STOCKS
DONATION	RECEIPT	TAXES

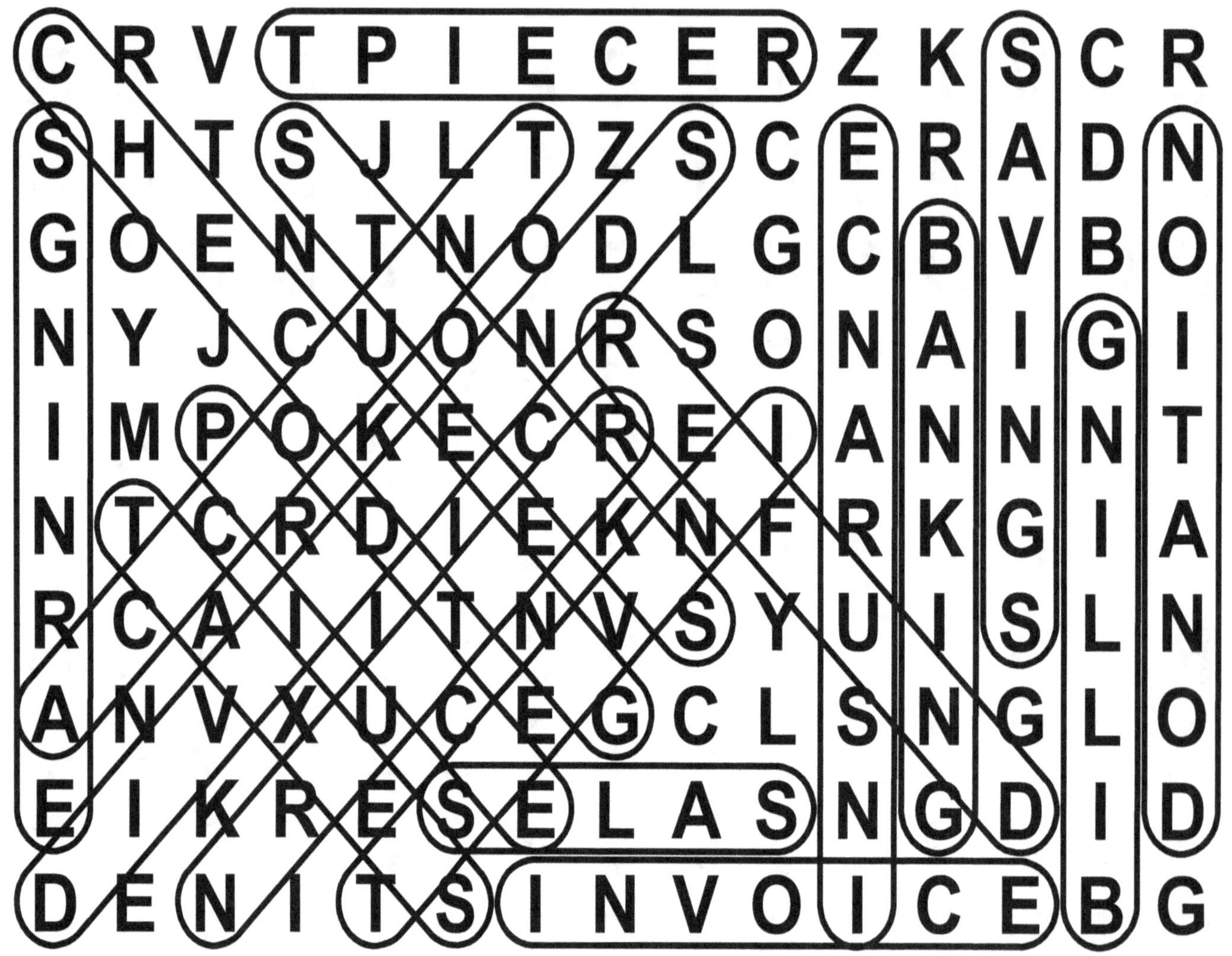

"Age is only a number we count until we're old enough to know it doesn't count."

~ Katrina Mayer

FAMOUS AUTHORS

```
R A X U S Y Q G K E R O U A C
E Y I W Y T C N N P O S M H G
N G E W D C O I E F E D L I W
K S N P I H N L T Q Q M L O B
L L R I C R R W S W O O L F R
U T E C K I O O U T U L E J E
A W V L E S Y R A D O R W O L
F A J Q N T P K F Q Z Y R Y I
X I J I S I A W A H S O O C A
J N P G J E I E L L I V L E M
```

AUSTEN	KEROUAC	SHAW
CHRISTIE	KING	TOLSTOY
CONROY	MAILER	TWAIN
DICKENS	MELVILLE	VERNE
FAULKNER	ORWELL	WILDE
JOYCE	ROWLING	WOOLF

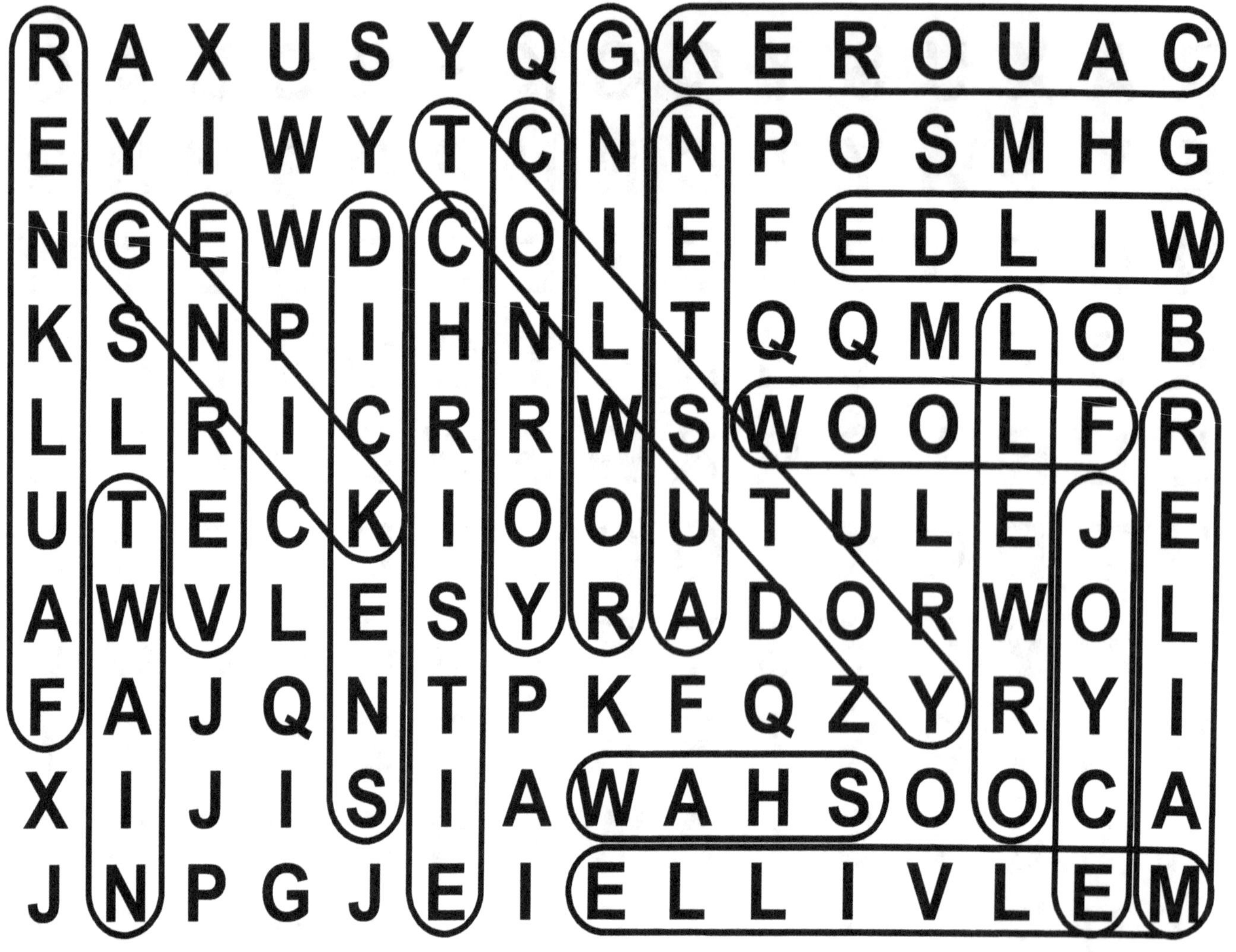

"That's the thing about books. They let you travel without moving your feet."

~ Jhumpa Lahiri

FOUR SEASONS

```
E N I H S N U S U M M E R A
M L P T M C H V R U L T H O
G Y K U S H O W E R S S H H
L W T F W I N T E R W E A T
E U W A U L W S G Q A R R R
A G O Q E L Y E H Q R N V I
D R N L Z Y X U H O M P E B
L E S A H E T I H W T J S E
O E N Q R U G N I R P S T R
C N R F L O W E R S M D E D
```

AUTUMN	HOT	SPRING
CHILLY	ORANGE	SUMMER
COLD	REBIRTH	SUNSHINE
FLOWERS	REST	WARM
GREEN	SHOWERS	WHITE
HARVEST	SNOW	WINTER

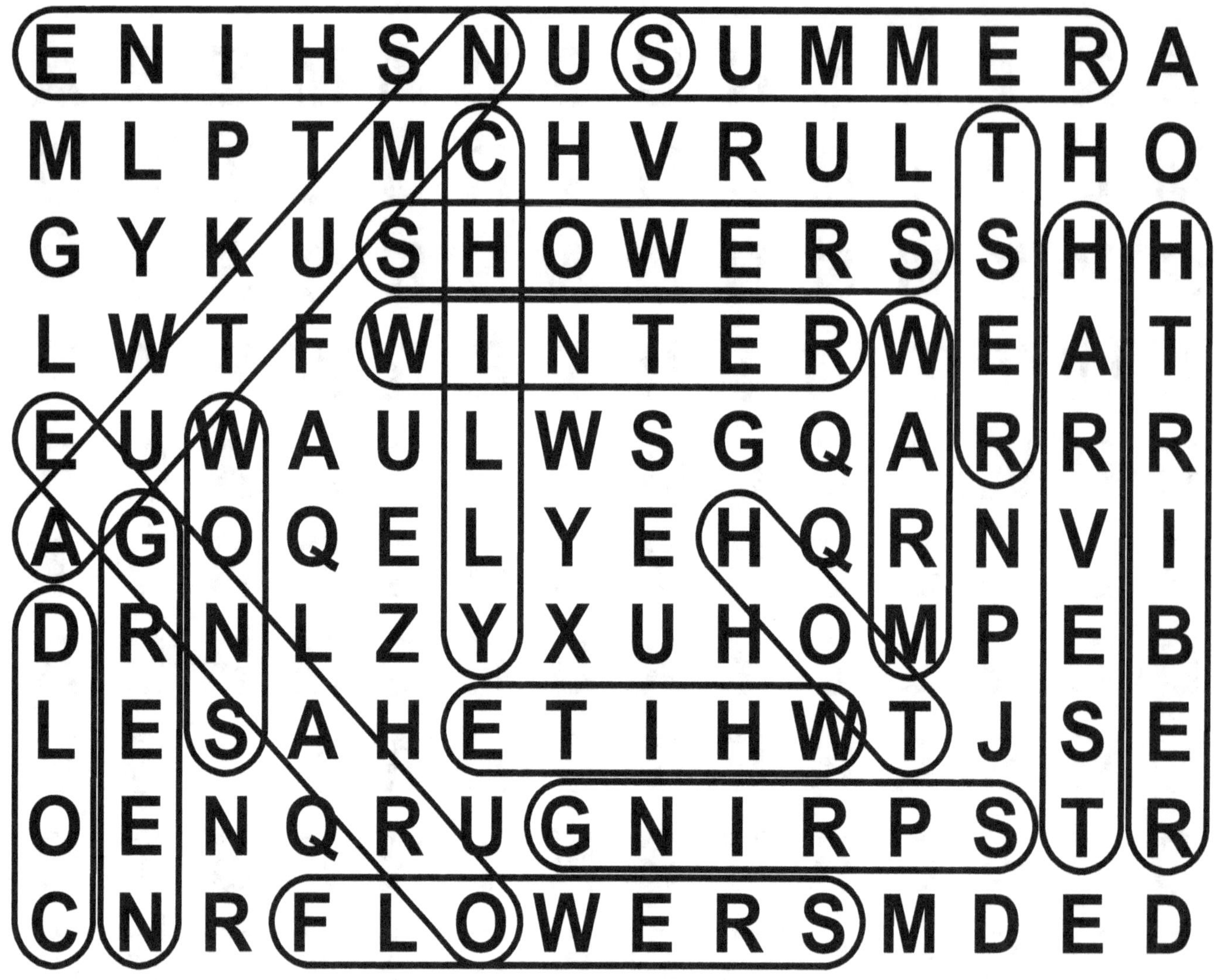

"For everything there is a season, and a time for every matter under heaven."

~ Ecclesiastes 3:1

I LOVE PUZZLES

```
F I G U R E Y S R K H D O W N
X L A J N O R K G E Y C V W B
N G E N U M B E R S W O T S X
E I R T S A D T Z S B S O A S
N A L L T Z S W L G D D N E M
I L F L O E F E S S O R C A F
F Y Z M I G R L U K O V O K Z
E I D I I F I S U L L L T W K
D A N S E A R C H J C X V J J
K N D D J I G S A W U C Y E I
```

ACROSS	FILL IN	MAZE
ANSWER	FIND	NUMBERS
CLUES	JIGSAW	SEARCH
DEFINE	LETTERS	SODOKU
DOWN	LOGIC	SOLVE
FIGURE	MATCH	WORDS

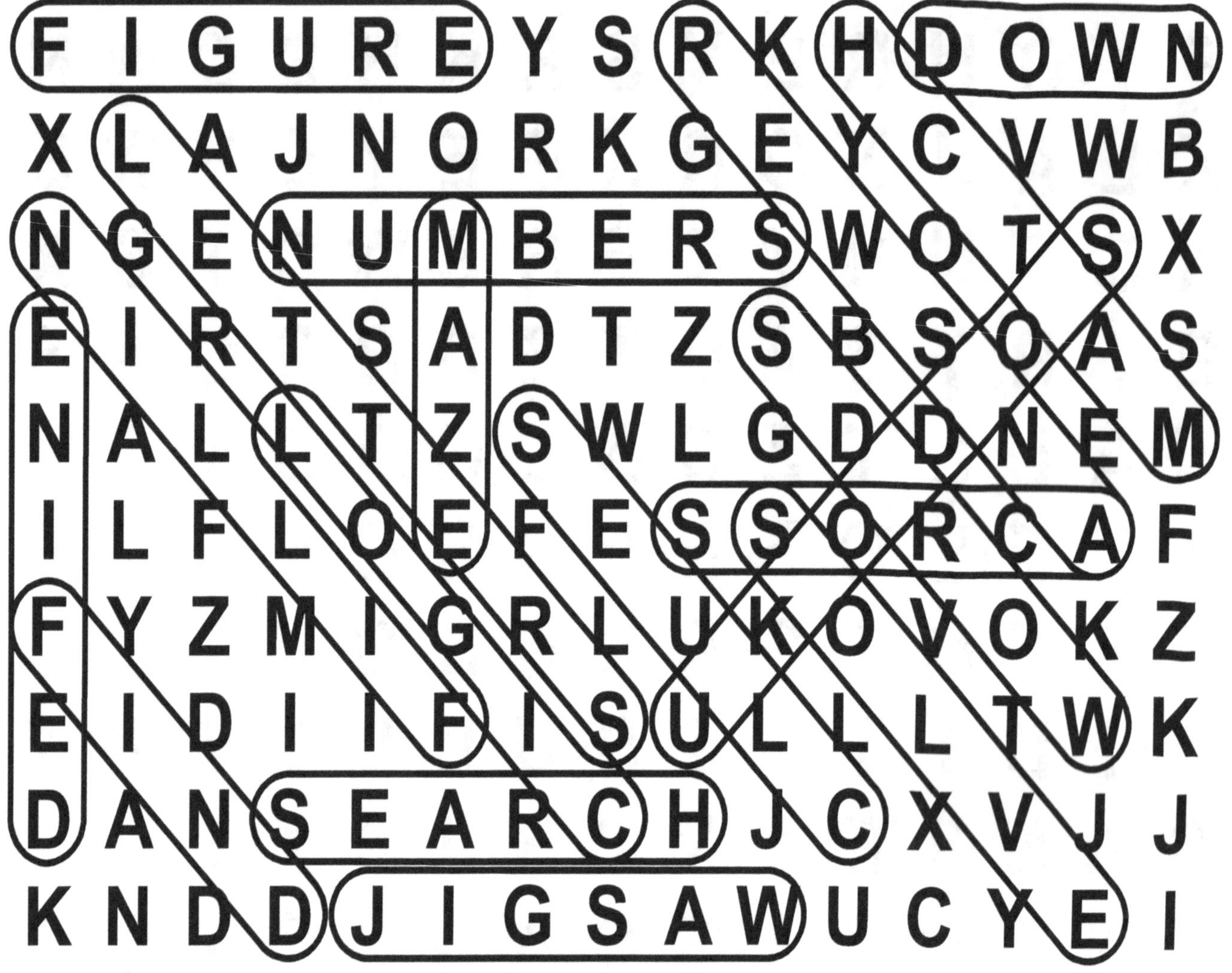

"God is putting the puzzle
of my life together."

~ Phillipians 1:6

IN THE LAB

C T Z N O I T U L O S R P A D
E L E M E N T S I T N E I C S
W S K S V S J A S E L G G O G
B K S U T S E E O S G N O T V
E S O A C T T R L C G L J K F
A K A A L T U O U S B G V L J
K T L G E G Y B W T T A A J U
E E S P B U R N E R L S L N J
R T I Y B U N S E N K U E Z X
S P D T Y R T S I M E H C T O

BEAKERS	FLASK	SCALE
BUNSEN	GAS	SCIENTIST
BURNER	GLASS	SOLUTION
CHEMISTRY	GOGGLES	TESTS
CULTURES	LAB COAT	TESTTUBE
ELEMENTS	PIPETTE	TONGS

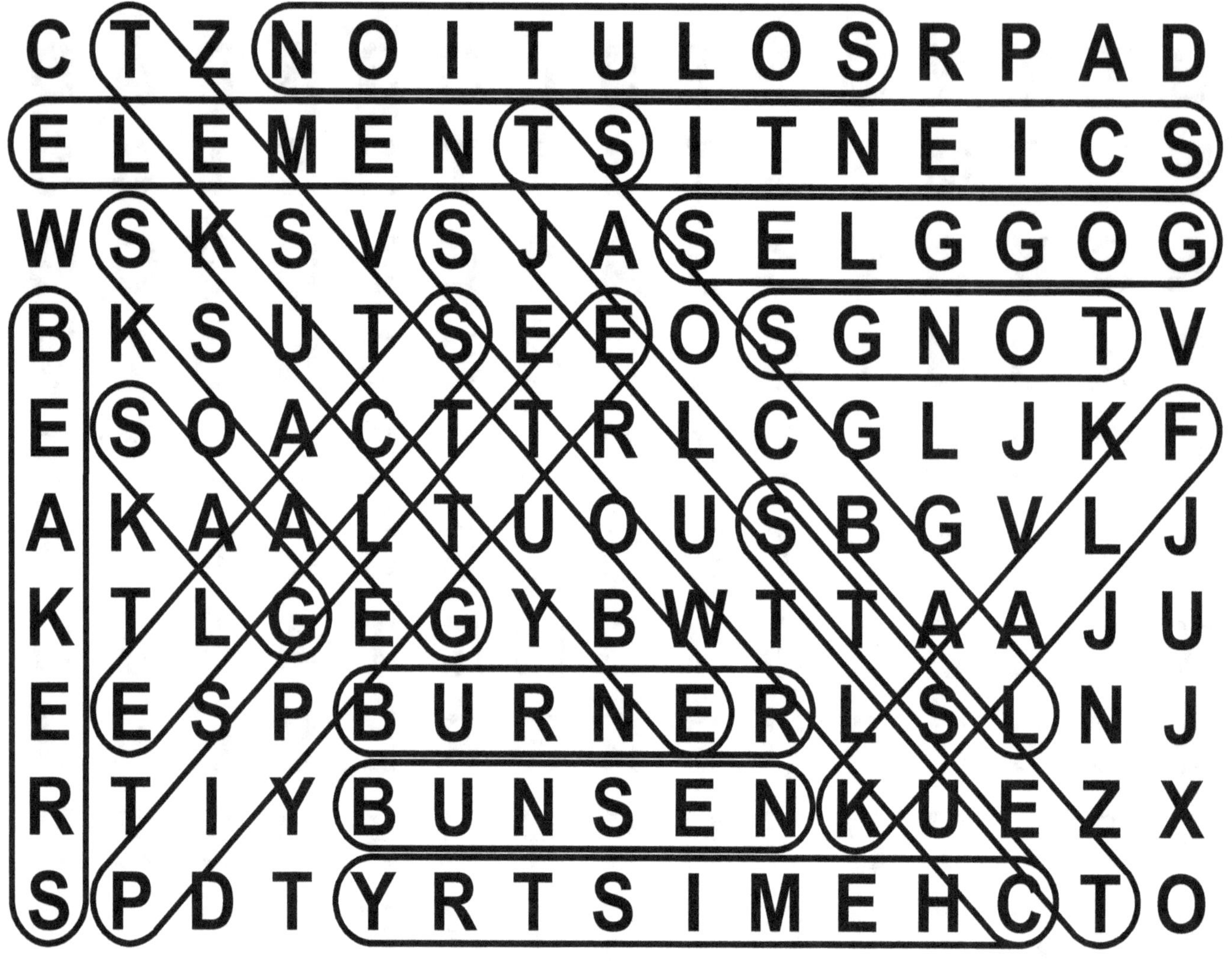

> "All the world is a laboratory
> to the inquiring mind."
>
> ~ Martin H. Fischer

IN THE RAINFOREST

```
G E Y G X B S Y G O L O C E T
K E T Y C G O Y S H R S W R N
A R R A O H E R U T E M O S S
M U M R M K D N C E N P F O N
T T F R N I B H R H I A B X R
O S H O M S L T D C I T L R E
R I M U E R I C A E M D V P F
R O H N N A V L B I R D S H H
A M I X W I T C A N O P Y C Z
P V E K A N S N A C U O T V O
```

BIRDS	MOISTURE	RAIN
CANOPY	MONKEY	SNAKE
CLIMATE	MOSS	TOUCAN
FERNS	ORCHIDS	TREES
FROGS	PARROT	TROPICAL
HUMID	PLANTS	VINES

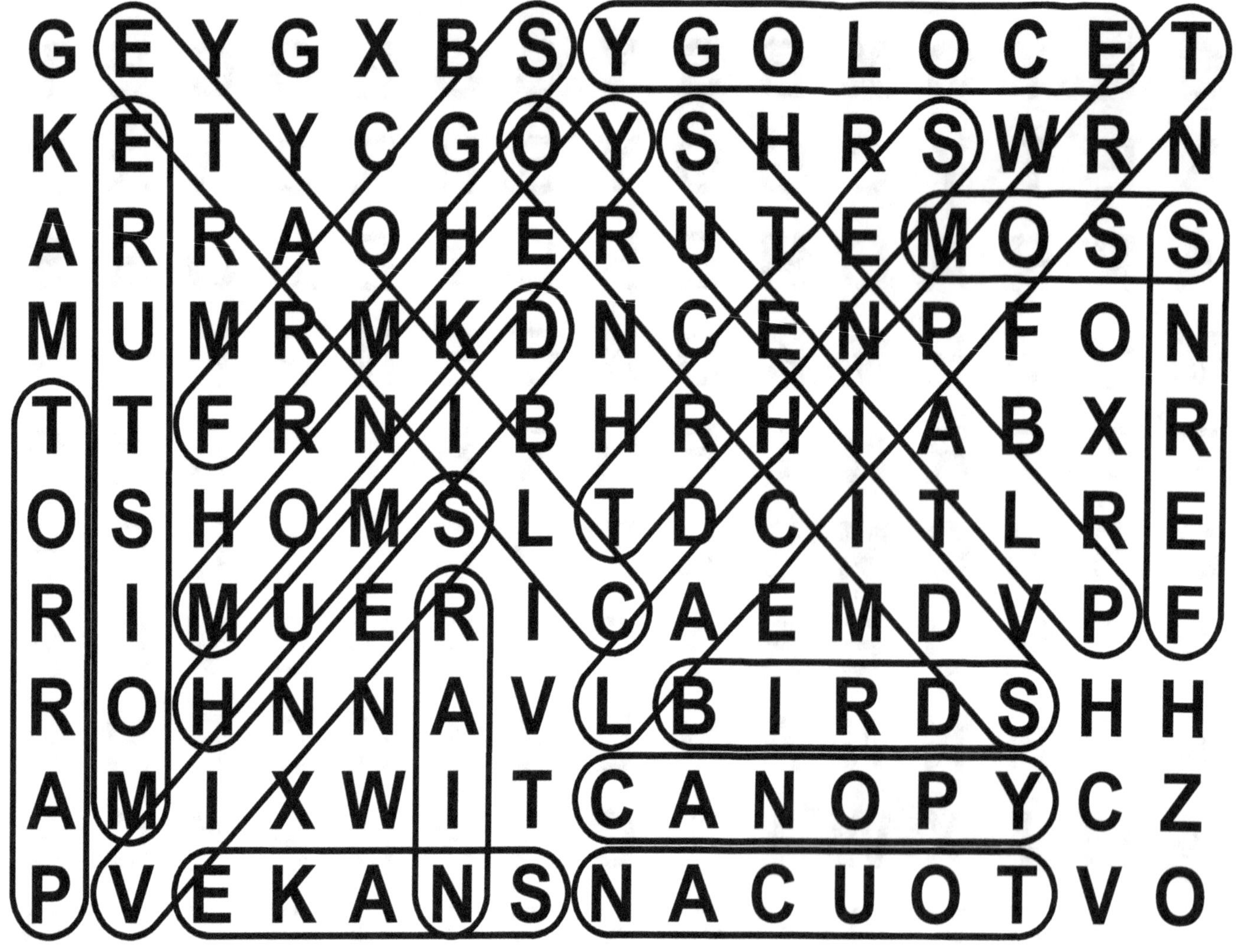

BONUS WORD TO FIND:

ECOLOGY

LET'S PLAY CARDS

```
D S H U F F L E K X H B J E S
I V S D F E G A B B I R C L K
S D I I S T R A E H T R D H C
C H F A Q E W I E F U F O C A
A U O M T G D J A M A C W O J
R E G D I R B A M T W T A N K
D E T L R N M Y P A I I R I C
S E K O L Q W Z R S P L D P A
P I S O C A N A S T A O O S L
Q Z R Q P V N N D E A L M S B
```

BLACKJACK	DRAW	ROOK
BRIDGE	GO FISH	RUMMY
CANASTA	HEARTS	SHUFFLE
CRIBBAGE	OLD MAID	SOLITAIRE
DEAL	PINOCHLE	SPADES
DISCARD	POKER	WAR

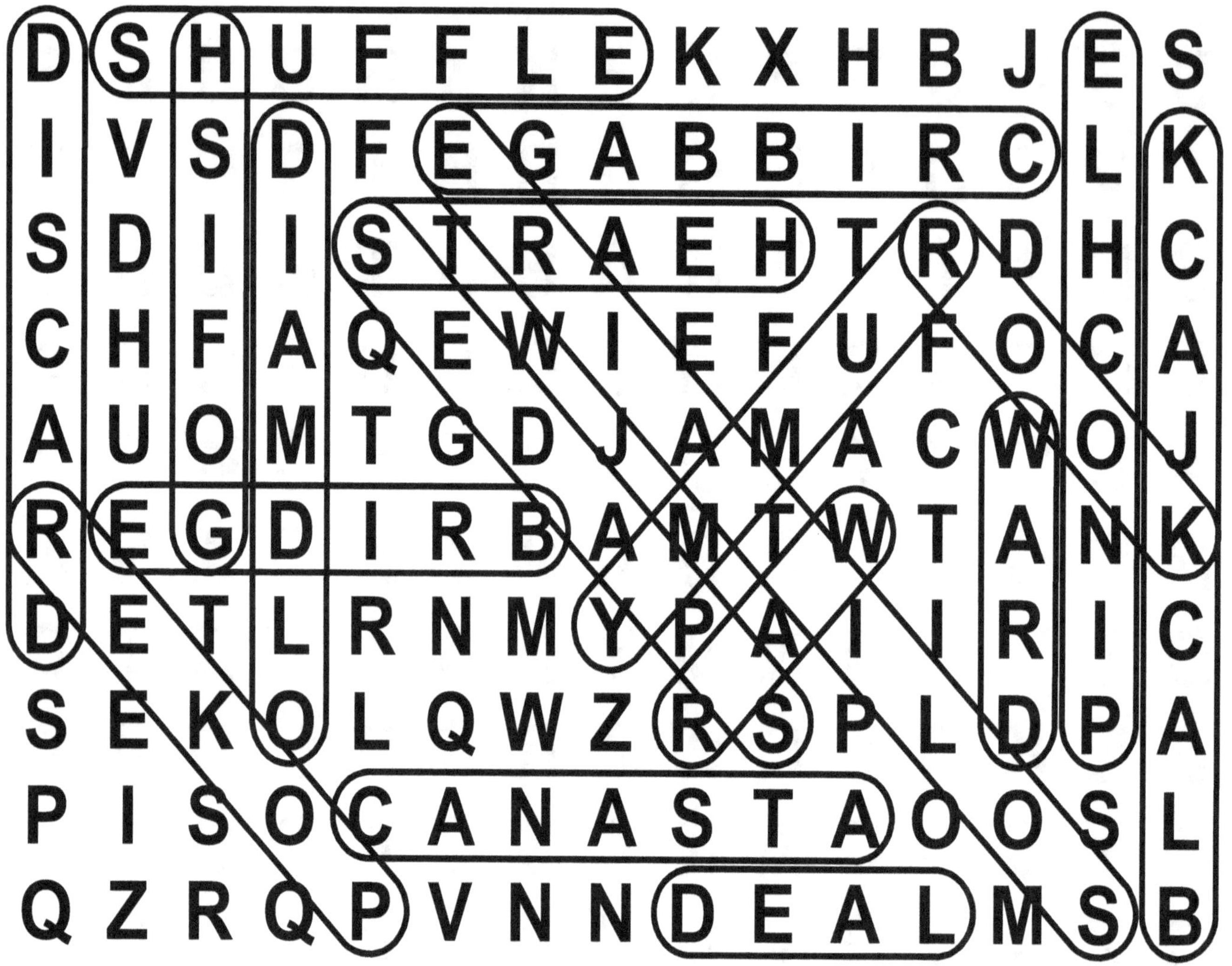

FUN FACT:

The first playing cards appeared in the 9th century during the Tang-dynasty in China.

PICNIC IN THE PARK

```
E N I H S N U S Q C U K X W E
C E D M H B T S A B H H D I A
I Y A S I M R A H L J E L N E
N R E G A E S R U A G T E E T
C G R A P N P G B N E N M S D
I N B M I L D X X K Y T O P E
P U A K A D C W S E S T N A C
M H P T R U V A I T Q Z A R I
D A E N P B B G E C Y F D K M
N S I S O M R E H T H H E U S
```

ANTS	GRASS	PARK
BASKET	HAMPER	PICNIC
BLANKET	HUNGRY	PLATES
BREAD	ICED TEA	SANDWICH
CHEESE	LEMONADE	THERMOS
CUPS	NAPKINS	WINE

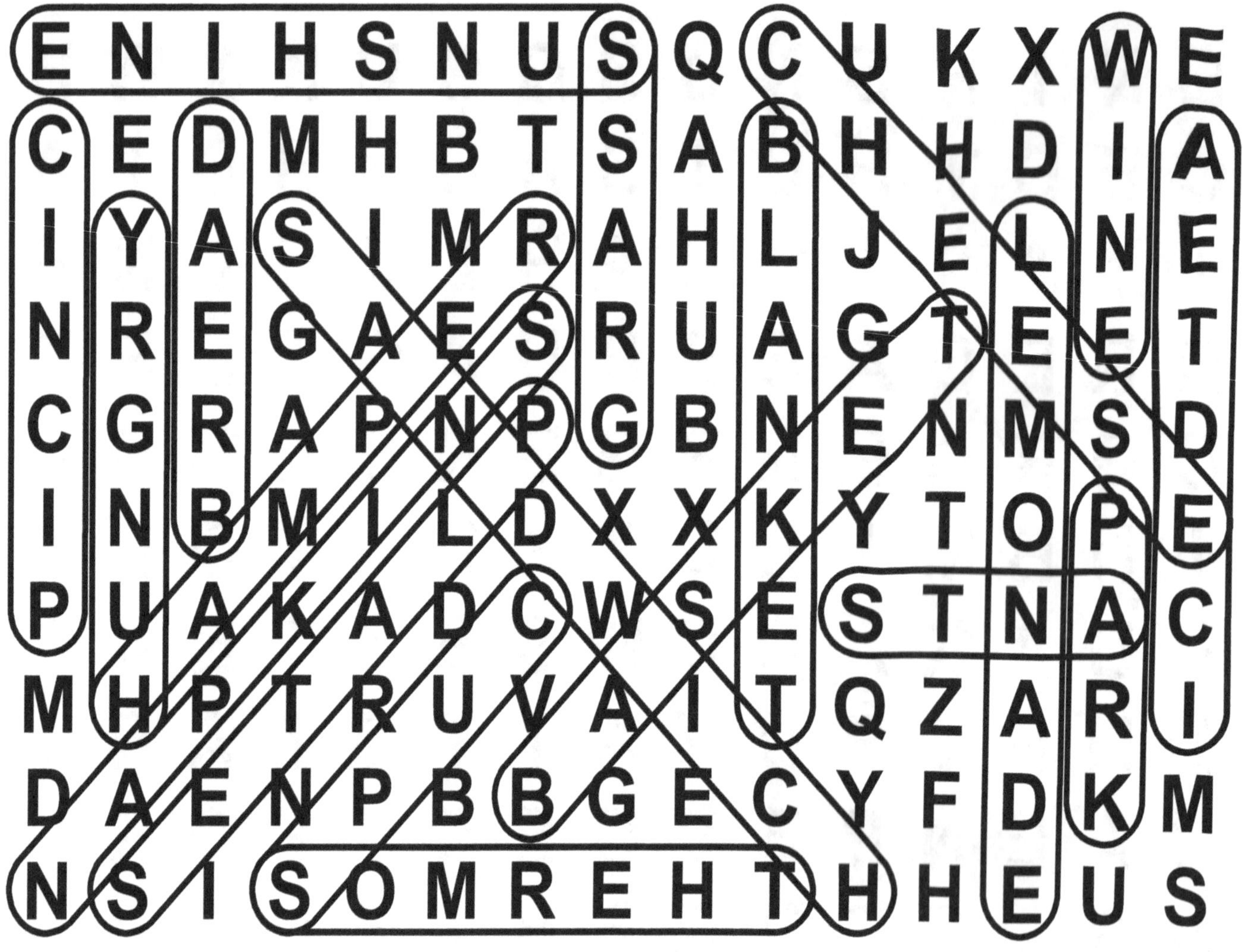

BONUS WORD TO FIND:

SUNSHINE

SO MANY BOOKS

```
A U T H O R S S N R I R E B E
M T E U E F P A R C S L Y E E
H N S M T I Y R A R B I L P R
A E O N O C S E R I E S U H U
D R M N N T C V B G T Z H I T
A Y G P G I H D X O Z N G S C
H Y T B V O O V R L U E C T I
R P B T D N O E E S B O U O P
W Y S E M U L O V P O E T R Y
D H H Y K C E H C K T G Y Y W
```

AUTHORS	LIBRARY	SCRAP
CHECK	NOTE	SERIES
COOK	PICTURE	STORE
FICTION	POETRY	TOME
HISTORY	PUZZLE	USED
HYMN	SCHOOL	VOLUMES

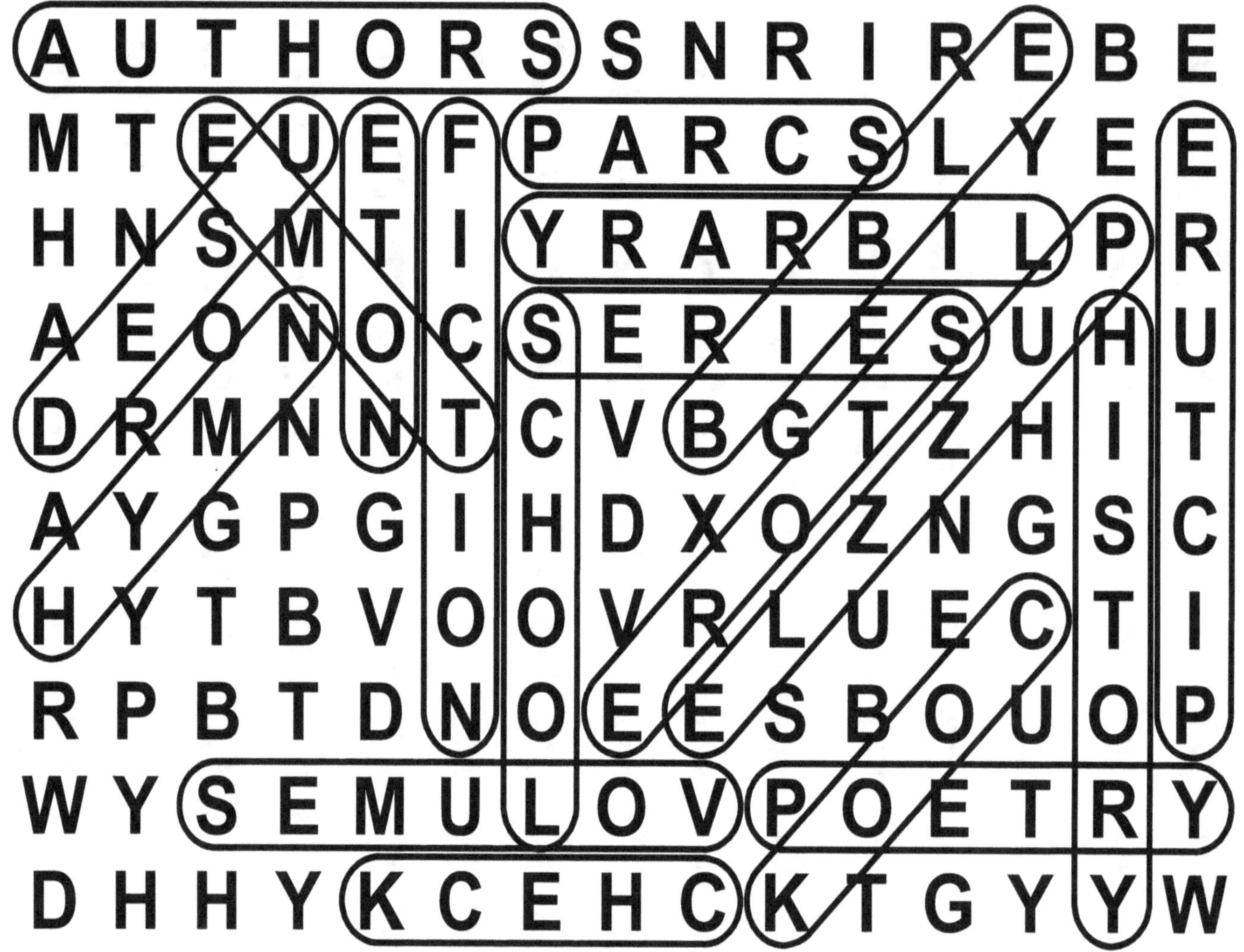

BONUS WORD TO FIND:

BIBLE

SPACE

```
S Z M M H T R A E R X W X Y D
T N N I C S U N A R U M A R S
E E R K L B U L W R S K N P N
M P U N L K O N E M Y R T L O
O T T P N S Y T E P S O I A O
C U A V V Y I W H V T C B N M
S N S O X P K A A W E K R E S
M E R C U R Y X B Y M E O T A
N X H J O W W P G P Y T M S W
T U B O T U L P M E T E O R S
```

COMETS	MILKYWAY	ROCKET
EARTH	MOONS	SATURN
JUPITER	NEPTUNE	SOLAR
MARS	ORBIT	SYSTEM
MERCURY	PLANETS	URANUS
METEORS	PLUTO	VENUS

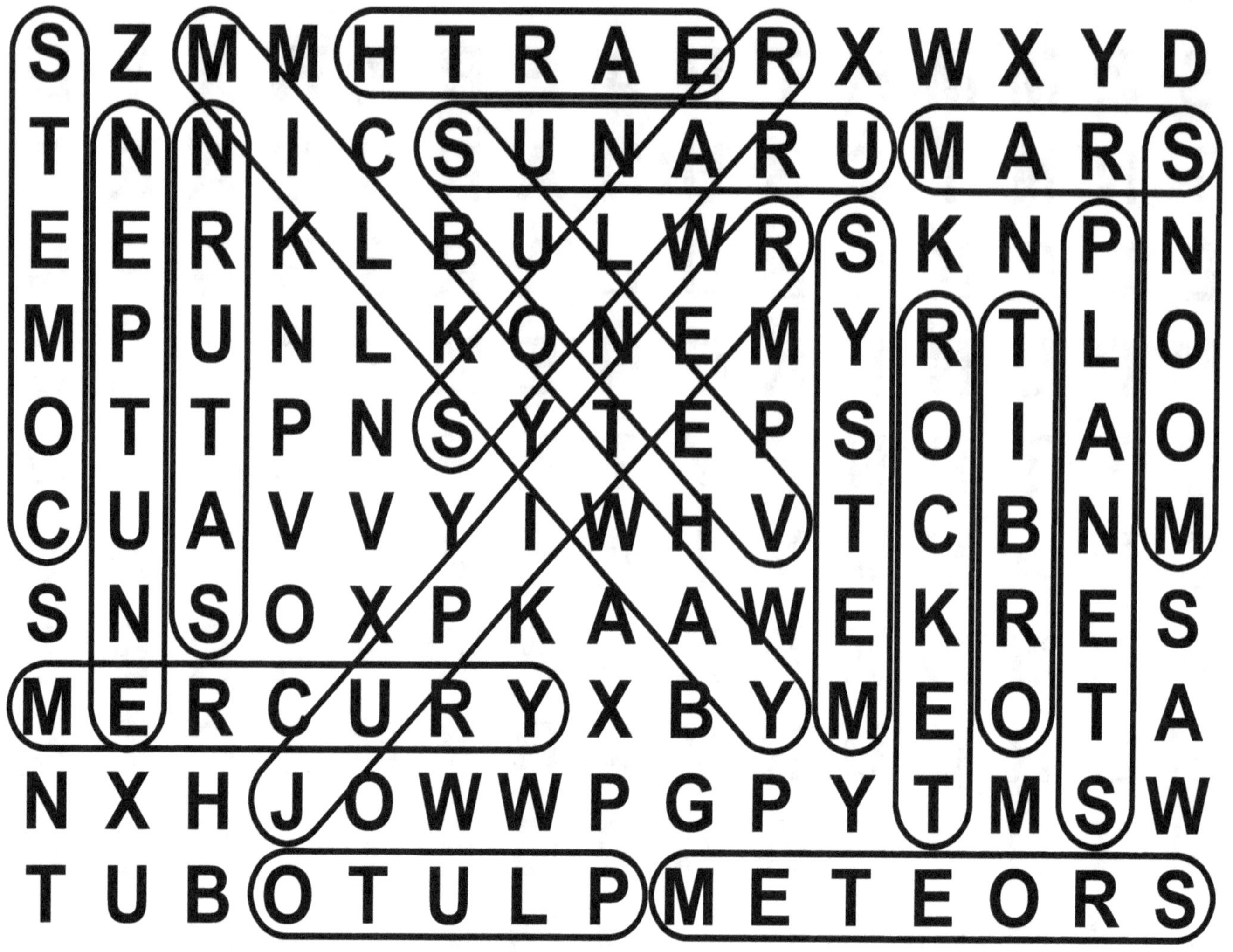

> "The heavens declare
> the glory of God"
>
> ~ Psalm 19:1

STARTS WITH P

```
J  H  P  I  E  C  E  G  L  D  P  P  U  L  L
T  E  V  R  E  S  E  R  P  U  P  O  P  U  P
N  Y  Q  Z  S  P  P  P  Z  I  P  L  E  T  E
E  P  W  B  S  R  I  Z  A  I  R  V  E  P  A
S  R  F  G  A  P  L  Z  N  I  I  E  R  P  C
E  U  H  I  P  E  I  G  Z  T  N  I  P  R  E
R  D  S  O  S  P  P  L  I  A  N  T  L  A  R
P  E  I  Y  S  O  U  S  L  T  Z  N  H  Y  P
R  N  C  C  N  H  O  S  G  O  U  Z  P  E  M
T  T  A  G  B  P  J  E  H  Q  W  W  B  R  C
```

PAINT	PIZZAZZ	PRESENT
PAPER	POINT	PRESERVE
PEACE	POPUP	PRINT
PIECE	POSITIVE	PRUDENT
PILLOW	PRAISE	PULL
PINGPONG	PRAYER	PUSH

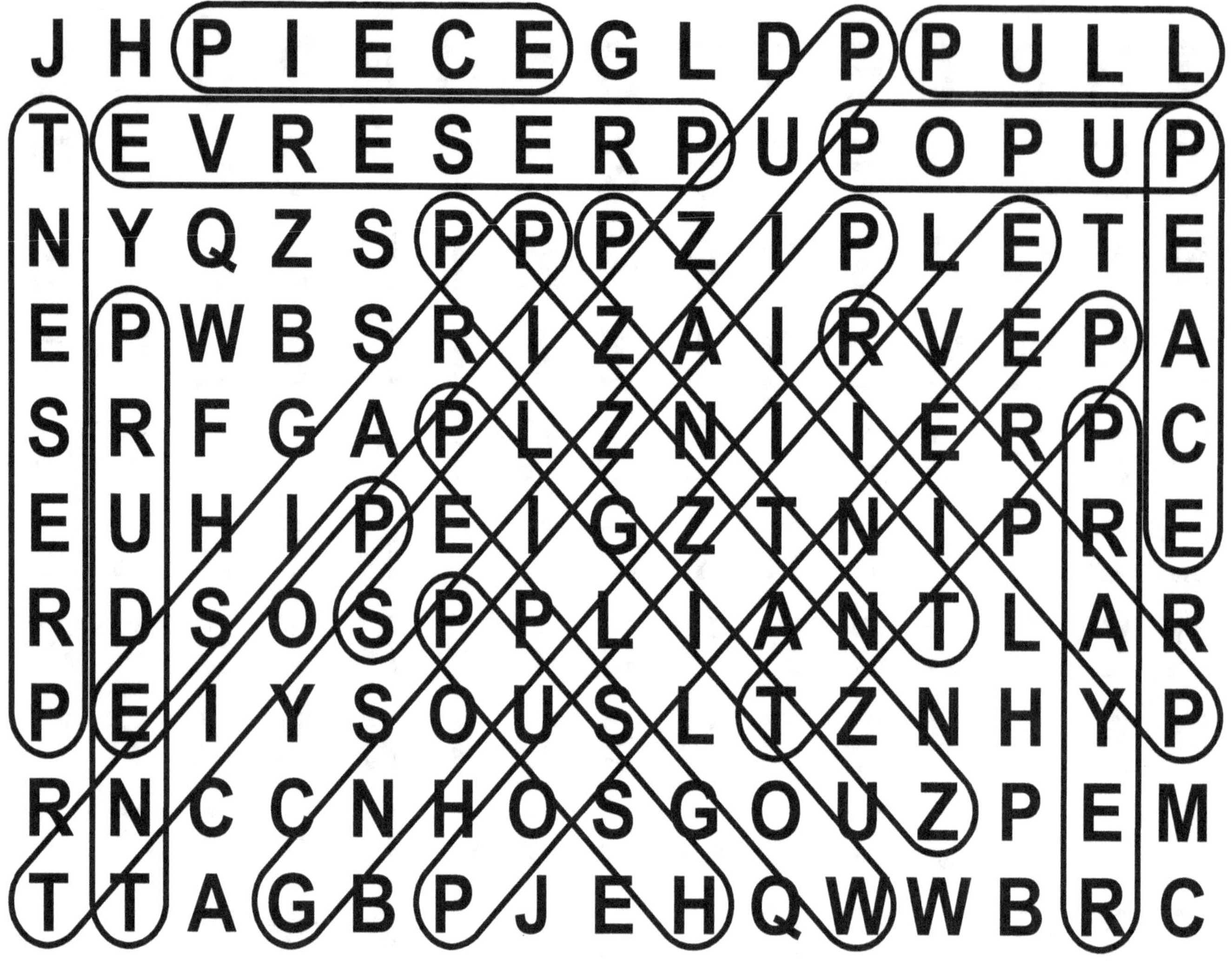

BONUS WORD TO FIND:

PUZZLES

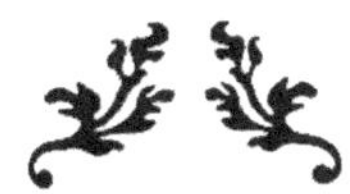

Number Search
Puzzle Section

Number Search puzzles are just like Word Search using a list of numbers instead of words.

The numbers can be forward, backward, up, down or diagonal, and may overlap.

Number Search #1

8 5 5 9 9 8 1 4 6 8 7 7 3 1
2 6 1 5 8 6 2 7 3 8 5 9 1 1
4 2 6 4 5 7 1 2 1 7 7 1 7 1
8 1 5 2 3 1 7 9 8 7 2 5 2 7
7 5 2 6 6 5 2 7 5 9 0 2 1 1
9 9 6 3 0 7 3 2 5 1 7 1 1 0
7 4 3 6 2 7 8 4 9 4 9 5 9 0
6 4 8 1 4 6 1 7 1 9 6 1 5 5
7 1 9 7 7 9 3 9 3 4 5 8 5 7
6 8 4 6 3 3 7 6 8 9 4 4 3 9

0057	4336	7590
1958	4599	7693
2177	5551	7876
2473	6626	8605
3534	6767	8773
3977	7474	9147

8 5 5 9 9 8 1 4 6 8 7 7 3 1
2 6 1 5 8 6 2 7 3 8 5 9 1 1
4 2 6 4 5 7 1 2 1 7 7 1 7 1
8 1 5 2 3 1 7 9 8 7 2 5 2 7
7 5 2 6 6 5 2 7 5 9 0 2 1 1
9 9 6 3 0 7 3 2 5 1 7 1 1 0
7 4 3 6 2 7 8 4 9 4 9 5 9 0
6 4 8 1 4 6 1 7 1 9 6 1 5 5
7 1 9 7 7 9 3 9 3 4 5 8 5 7
6 8 4 6 3 3 7 6 8 9 4 4 3 9

Number Search #2

```
5 5 1 0 2 8 4 5 4 8 8 6 2 1
5 7 2 5 6 7 2 3 8 3 9 3 7 1
3 0 8 0 1 9 9 1 6 0 9 4 5 2
5 5 7 3 0 7 9 3 3 3 2 4 6 1
7 3 5 5 3 4 7 0 8 7 2 9 5 7
9 4 4 6 9 0 5 9 5 7 3 3 2 7
4 4 2 6 4 3 2 1 2 2 9 6 4 5
3 2 4 4 3 6 8 0 8 8 9 7 1 1
4 4 5 8 2 6 4 9 2 8 6 1 4 5
9 6 5 6 7 7 7 2 8 5 3 7 5 6
```

0503	3375	5291
0910	3579	6094
1121	4226	7792
2443	5075	8213
2688	5241	9509
2698	5290	9880

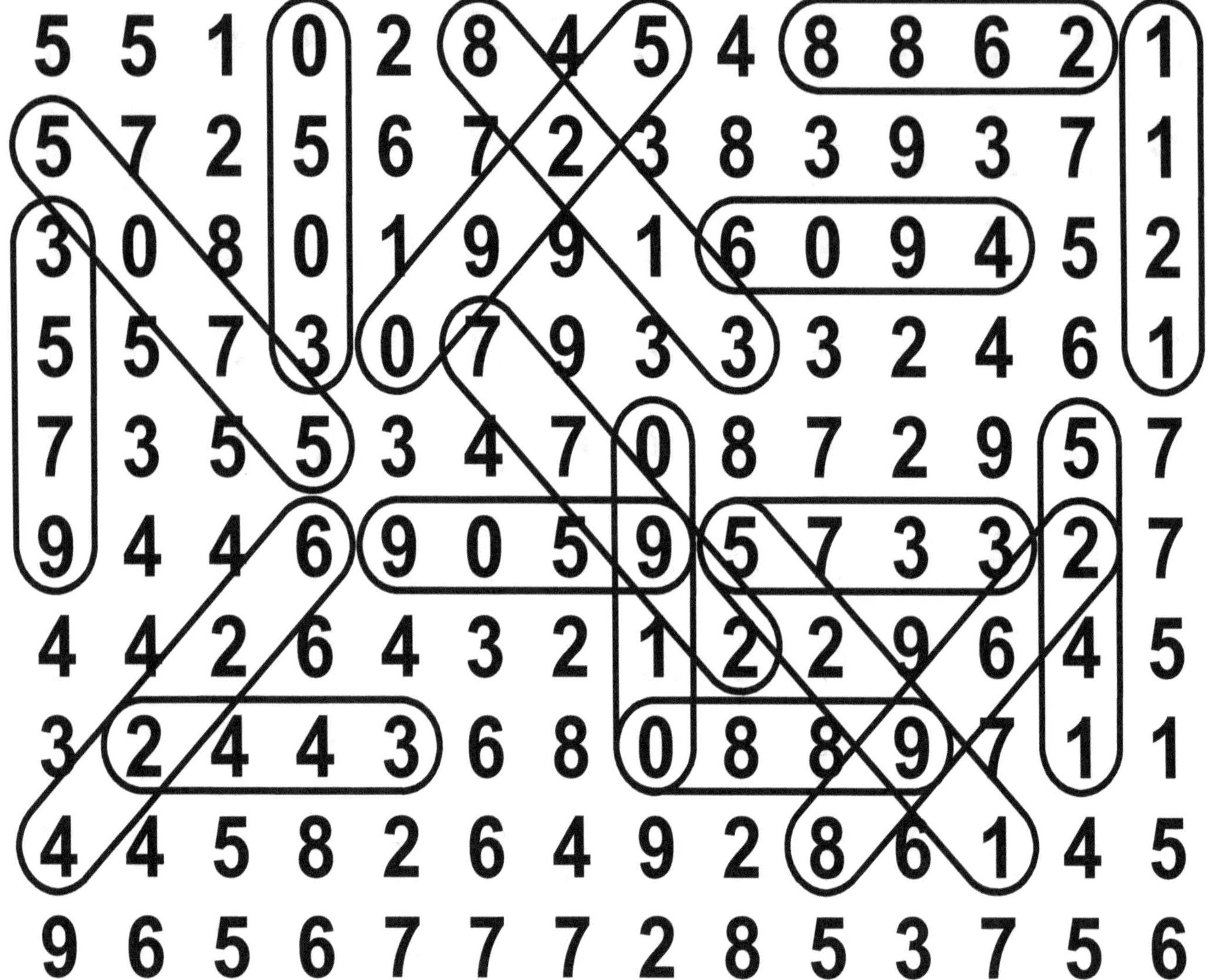

Number Search #5

```
1 9 4 3 6 3 7 3 1 9 3 5 3 4
6 5 1 5 0 5 3 1 8 5 9 2 4 7
4 1 1 1 6 4 9 2 3 5 6 2 2 3
3 5 0 0 7 7 5 5 6 6 7 8 7 8
7 0 4 0 7 9 0 2 0 3 9 5 9 1
1 8 1 0 7 5 3 3 1 6 2 7 2 6
7 1 1 5 3 2 6 6 2 5 4 8 9 0
3 9 1 1 2 9 7 4 6 7 7 0 7 7
8 8 0 0 6 4 3 6 3 6 7 9 3 8
4 4 4 7 8 1 9 3 6 0 6 5 8 4
```

01500	47613	64363
10010	56703	65701
22653	57520	70776
25975	59506	71153
37525	60639	95813
41110	63491	97243

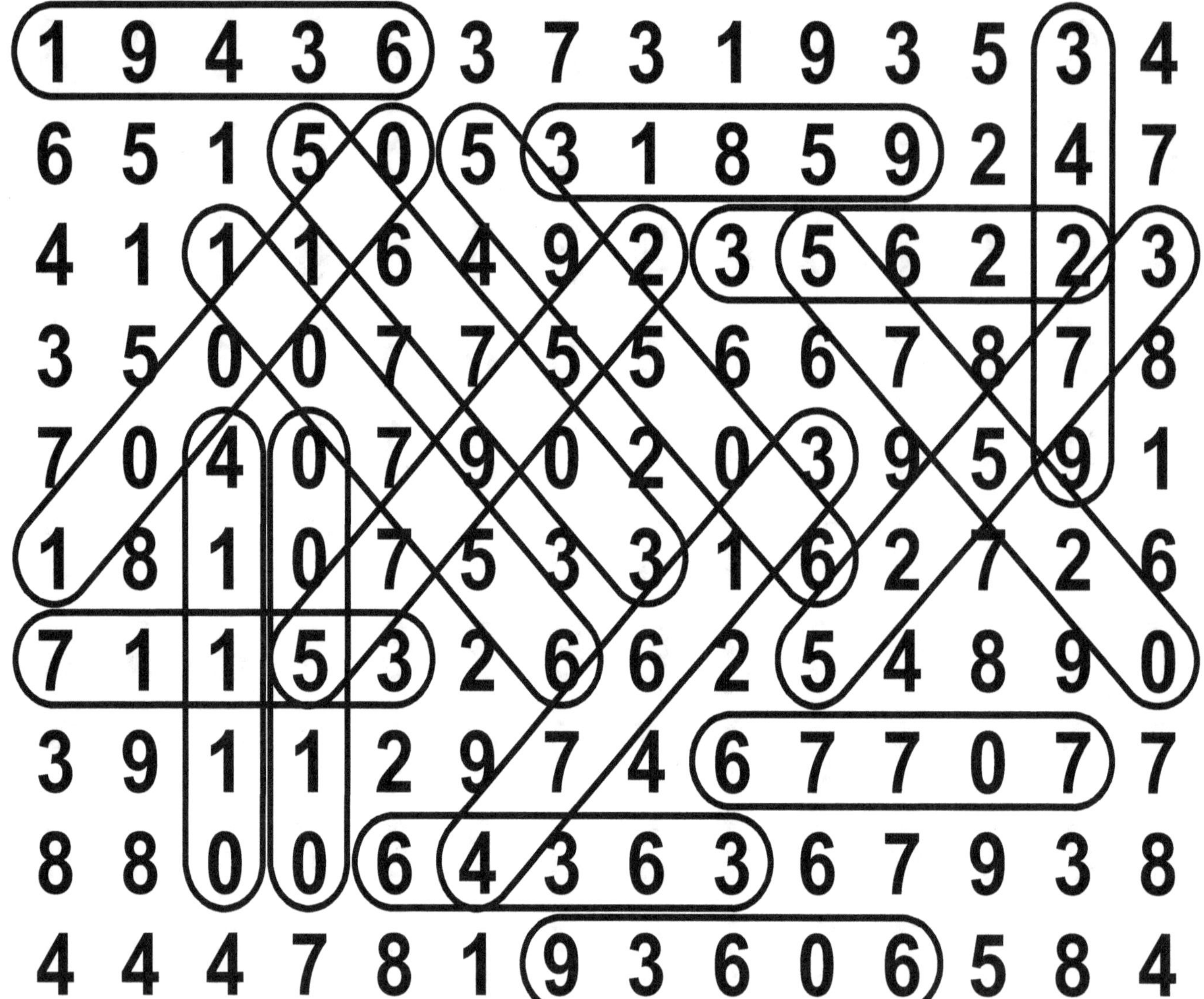

Number Search #6

5 8 1 5 2 7 9 6 2 4 6 3 0 4
3 2 2 8 3 4 2 2 9 6 9 2 8 8
2 8 6 3 2 9 5 3 9 7 2 3 4 8
2 1 9 0 1 2 4 7 5 4 2 5 7 9
3 8 6 9 8 1 8 1 2 5 2 7 8 2
0 3 1 3 2 7 6 1 3 5 1 2 3 5
8 1 8 5 0 8 4 8 9 6 1 4 2 8
5 5 0 2 7 8 9 9 7 8 2 6 5 7
1 9 5 6 6 8 8 9 7 6 7 2 5 2
5 5 2 6 4 5 6 2 6 9 3 0 7 6

03962	48892	63295
11732	50816	72112
24630	51580	81850
28613	52767	92899
35266	58526	93412
36786	58995	94780

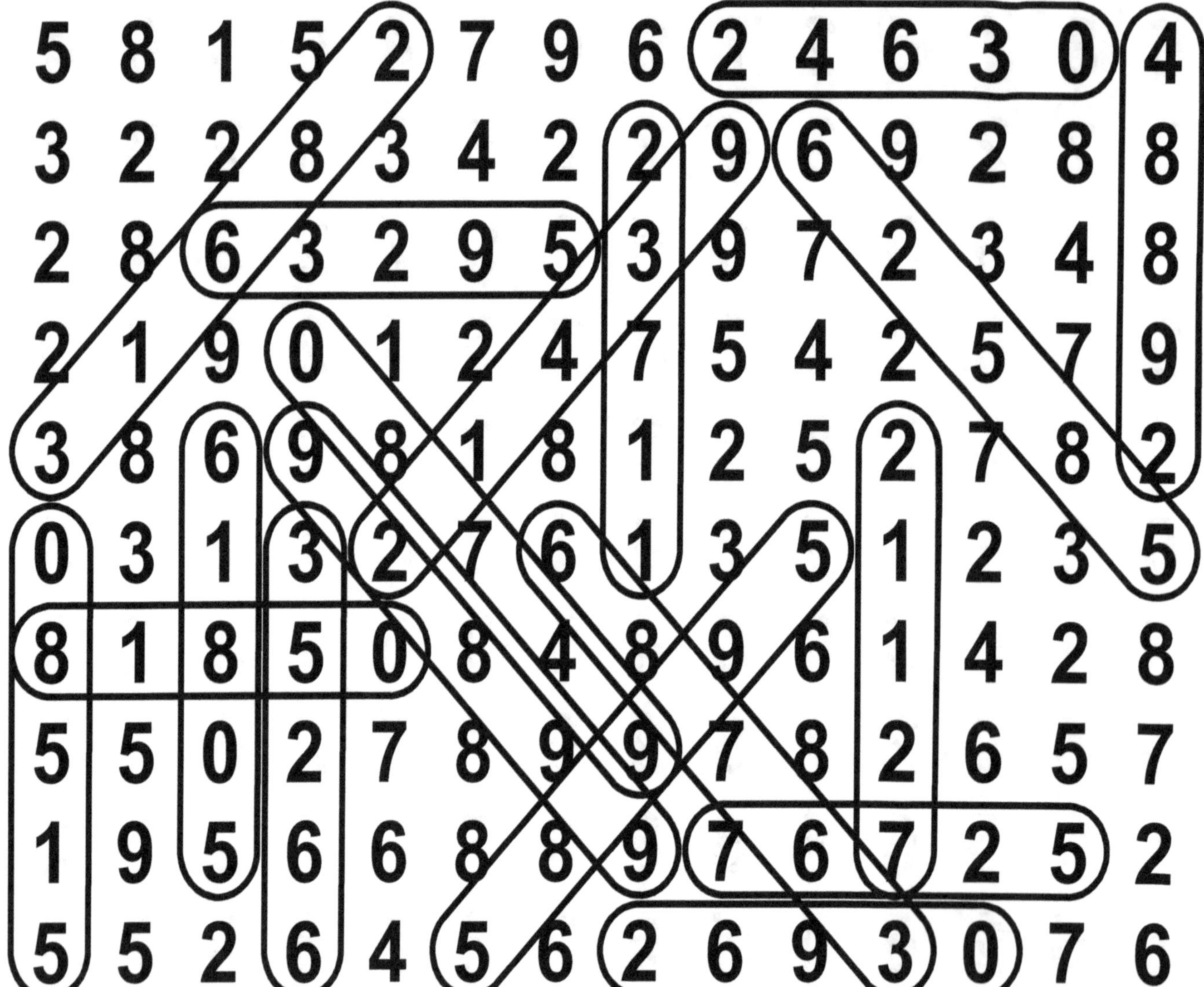

Number Search #7

```
7 6 8 6 2 4 9 4 5 1 8 6 3 1
7 8 2 9 1 3 5 4 7 8 9 7 9 5
6 2 3 7 3 7 5 2 1 2 5 5 9 7
5 7 4 3 5 7 0 0 3 6 0 8 6 4
8 9 7 8 9 3 1 2 2 8 2 5 0 6
9 4 7 1 8 7 4 8 3 1 8 6 1 0
8 0 4 7 5 3 6 5 6 7 4 1 1 6
2 5 6 5 1 3 3 1 5 8 3 6 5 2
3 0 8 0 4 8 2 2 6 2 1 5 4 5
8 1 5 1 6 5 9 4 0 3 9 9 6 0
```

01463	36086	57408
06250	40648	75347
20285	41749	81749
20532	47656	87608
26867	54512	98567
28408	54789	99304

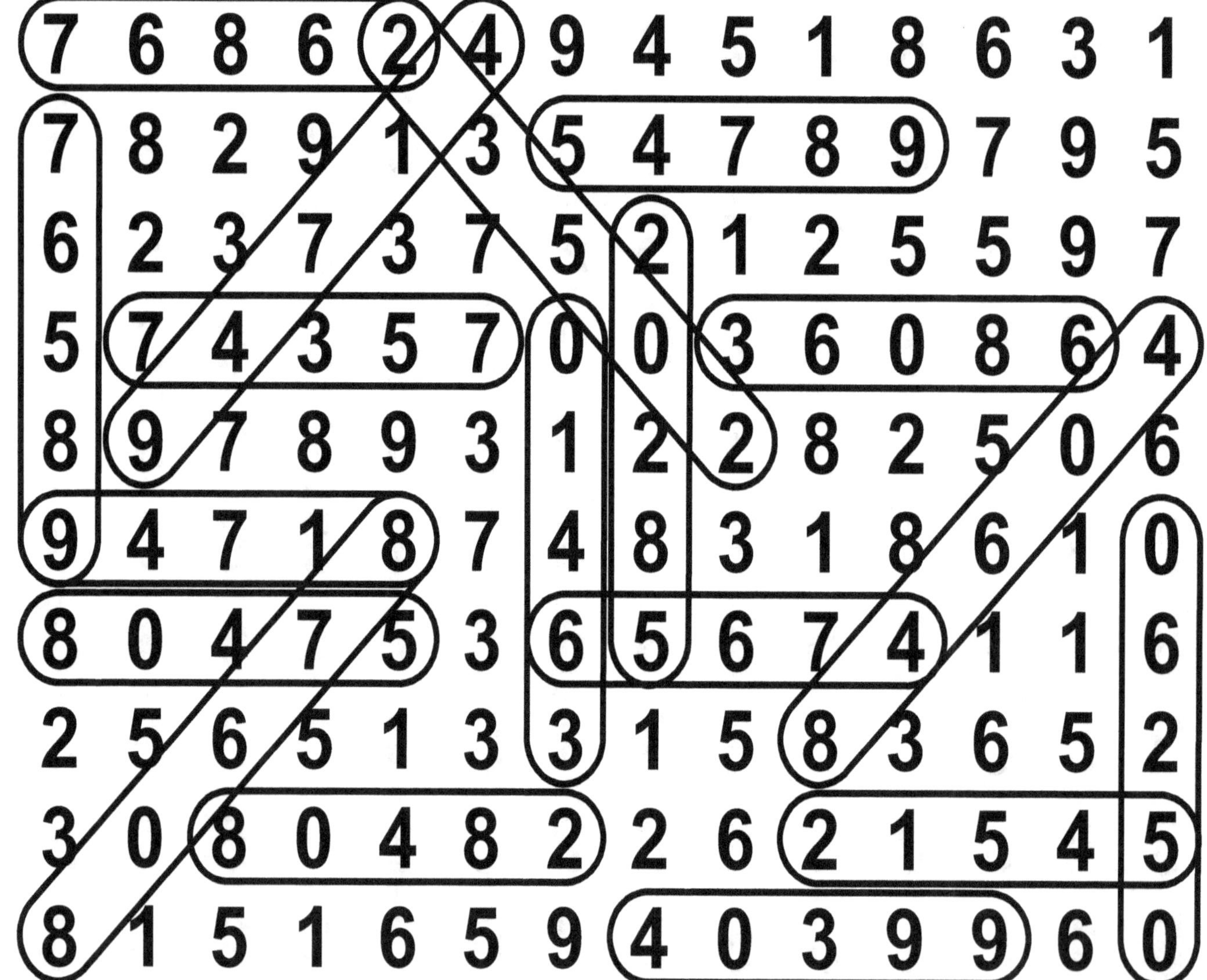

Number Search #8

7 3 5 6 4 7 2 4 4 8 9 6 1 7
2 3 9 5 9 2 9 5 9 6 2 5 3 9
8 2 8 1 5 7 9 4 6 0 8 1 3 1
8 8 5 7 7 6 4 5 9 3 9 3 5 0
7 4 0 0 7 2 4 1 5 8 7 2 1 2
8 1 8 2 3 5 3 5 0 9 7 6 0 2
9 6 7 6 6 7 4 6 1 8 4 6 7 2
2 7 4 2 0 3 8 2 6 7 4 0 5 8
8 2 3 3 7 6 5 6 9 3 5 8 5 3
5 6 2 2 3 9 8 7 7 9 5 5 1 6

06497	36860	80589
16984	52672	80662
26807	62239	82337
28302	65693	91548
31980	73190	95516
35107	79102	95962

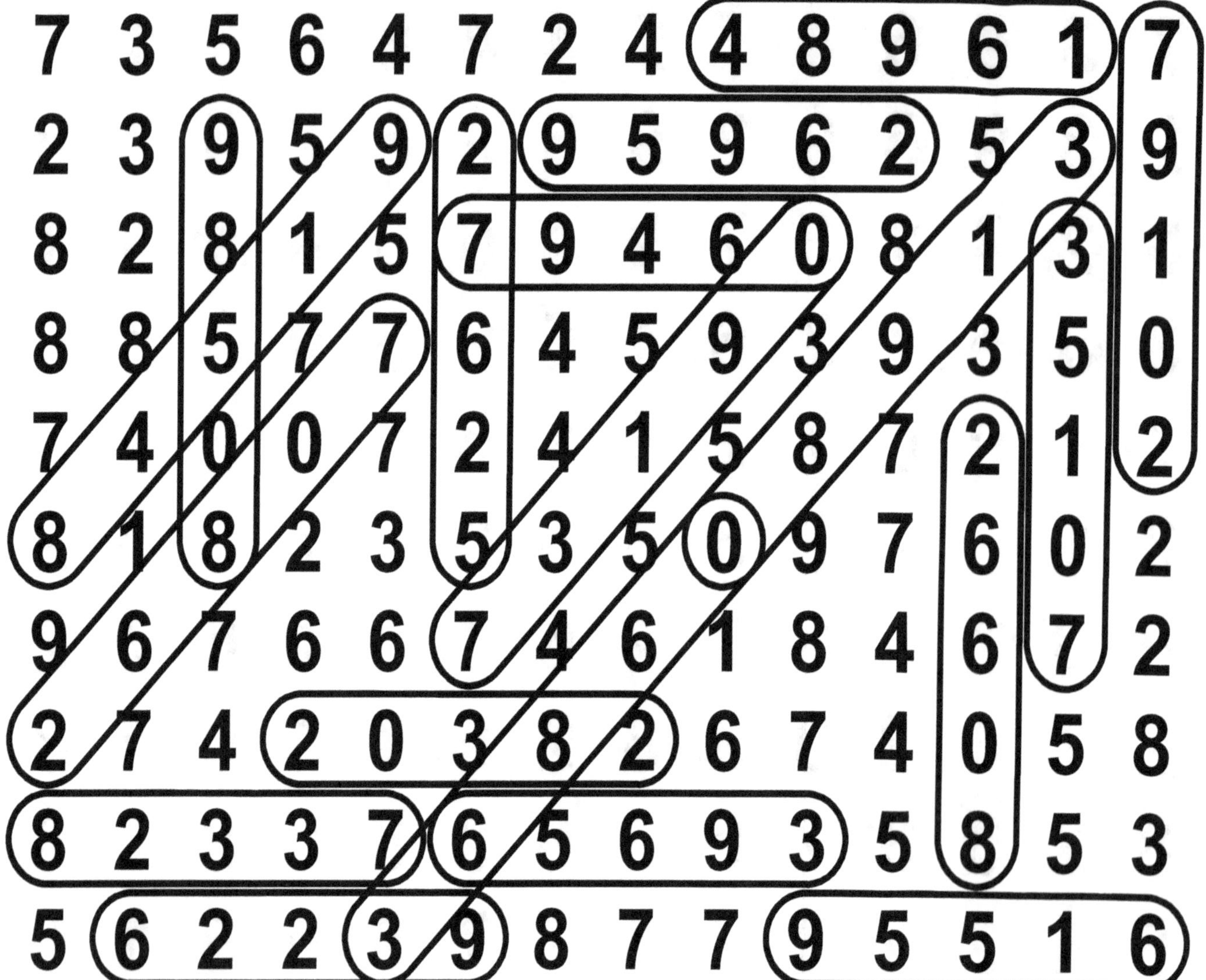

Number Search #9

9 3 7 1 5 0 4 3 5 4 1 5 5 6
7 6 5 4 9 1 3 6 6 9 7 2 8 8
9 4 3 2 6 5 4 6 5 1 7 7 3 8
8 5 1 8 7 6 1 1 0 4 5 8 4 5
8 3 9 9 3 8 5 3 1 1 9 6 0 6
9 0 1 2 6 2 1 2 9 6 0 4 1 3
9 9 1 6 7 5 0 1 3 3 3 4 3 6
9 5 9 3 1 1 4 3 4 3 3 6 3 4
3 8 3 1 8 6 3 8 2 8 1 4 4 7
9 0 7 7 2 9 8 7 6 6 6 6 6 9

015143	569147	834013
103151	669728	864464
141633	746365	876666
317295	781148	907729
330957	831616	931290
551453	832032	983108

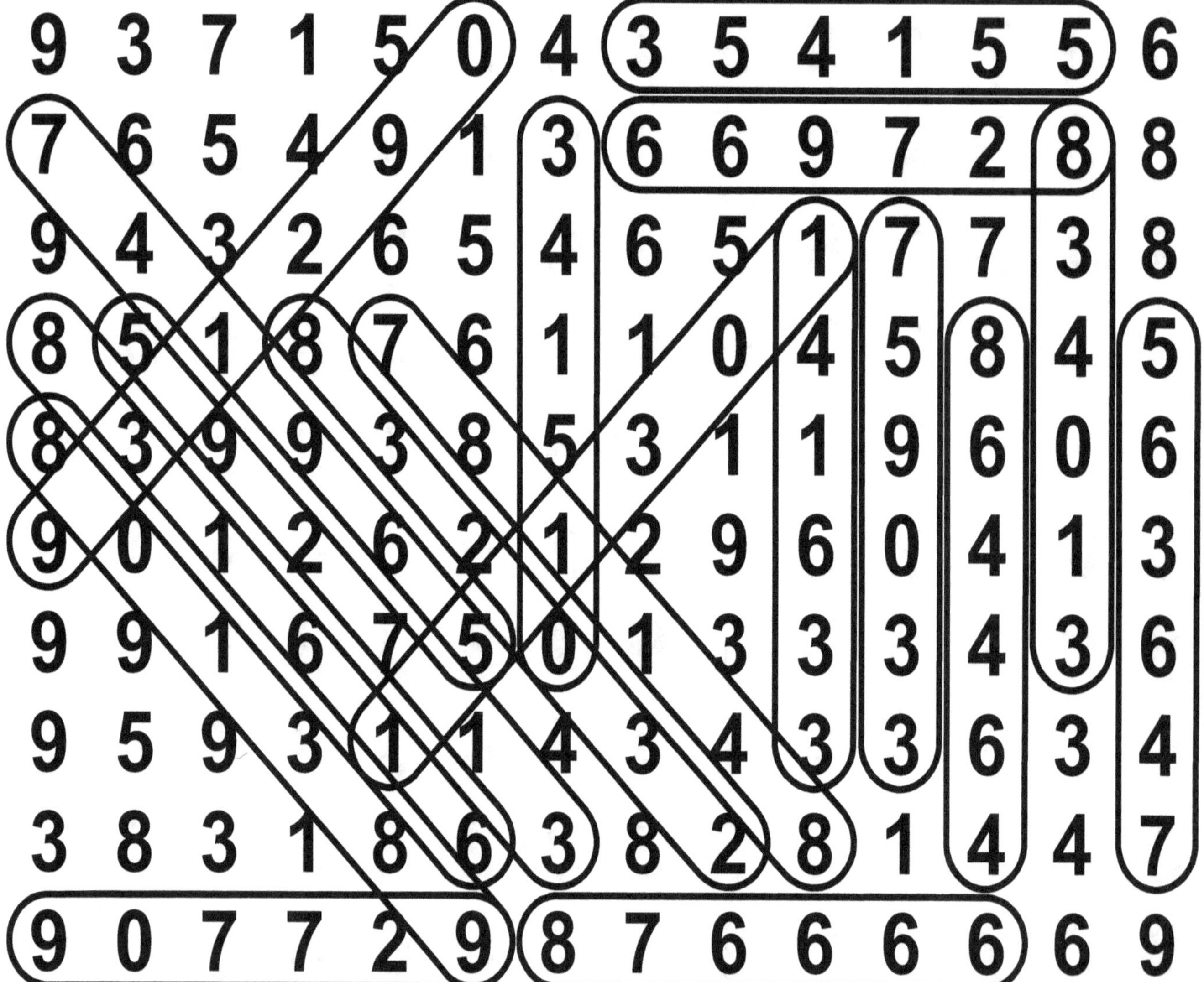

Number Search #10

```
9 2 8 3 8 1 5 6 8 9 2 5 5 7
4 7 5 4 2 5 3 9 2 3 2 6 2 5
9 3 6 7 6 1 0 5 3 9 5 6 7 0
8 2 7 1 5 8 1 2 5 9 8 6 1 1
6 3 4 2 8 3 1 8 7 8 3 1 6 3
3 5 4 4 8 3 8 1 5 4 4 0 0 9
2 9 7 6 7 9 0 1 6 1 7 4 5 1
6 0 1 1 4 9 2 3 4 6 2 5 4 5
7 6 6 7 8 3 5 7 8 8 3 2 1 9
4 5 0 2 6 0 2 2 4 4 6 5 6 7
```

013915	401666	716054
039395	447160	761053
123887	450260	885123
224465	529865	901795
235906	618303	958894
337721	642174	986326

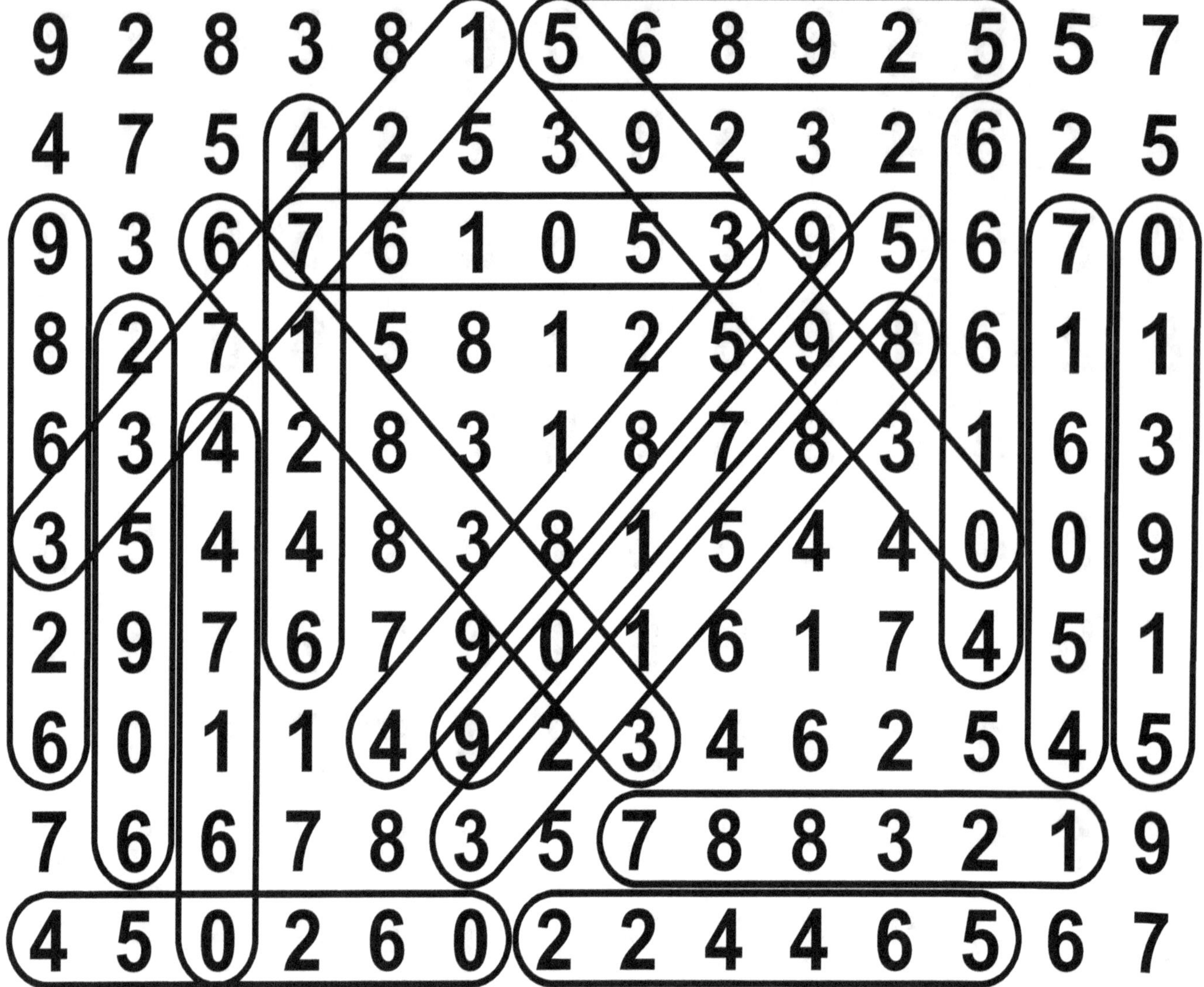

Number Search #11

3 2 2 3 6 8 1 1 2 1 9 4 7 3
8 3 2 3 2 2 8 1 7 5 9 9 8 0
8 4 2 5 6 9 7 4 3 7 8 3 3 6
8 3 2 9 2 1 8 3 8 1 7 9 2 9
0 3 3 7 6 9 8 3 6 4 1 9 1 7
8 3 1 3 4 5 5 3 1 0 3 7 9 3
8 3 9 8 1 1 9 6 4 5 2 7 3 7
8 7 6 5 7 4 3 7 1 1 6 4 1 5
5 4 5 4 8 2 4 7 7 7 7 3 2 5
8 2 3 8 2 2 6 1 8 0 0 3 1 2

112194	322368	737960
140517	329659	831563
171639	338515	848437
172171	482477	880888
213008	592522	884936
238226	733334	899571

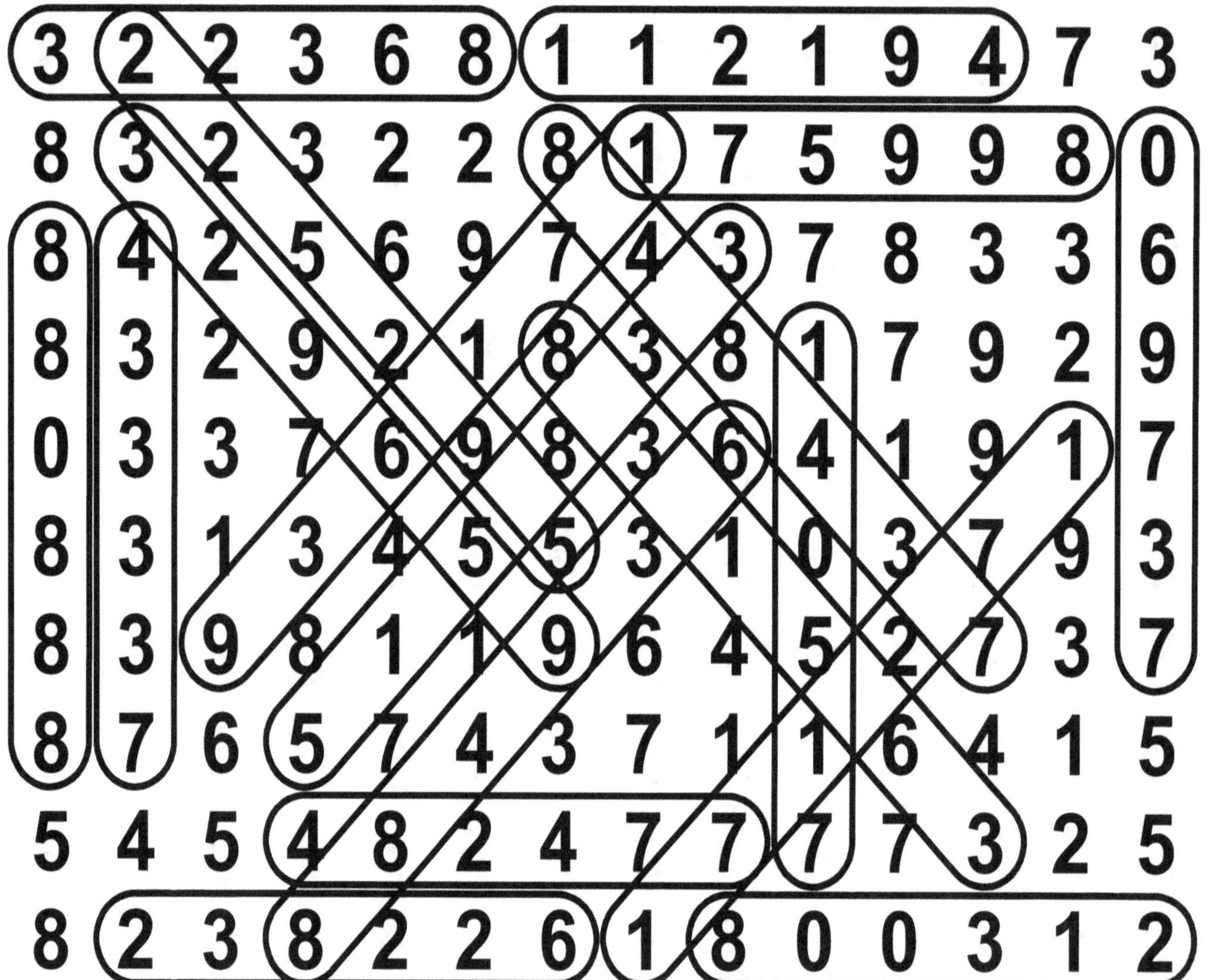

Number Search #12

1 7 2 5 4 2 9 9 8 8 2 2 8 4
8 2 9 3 3 5 0 7 8 8 8 4 1 9
5 6 8 2 4 1 3 0 3 7 6 9 5 4
1 9 2 5 9 8 8 3 4 8 8 6 7 5
7 1 9 3 9 2 9 8 2 8 8 0 9 4
3 5 9 2 9 1 6 9 4 1 5 2 8 4
2 4 6 9 9 0 1 7 2 6 5 1 4 1
7 0 7 6 9 0 4 3 7 7 5 9 4 2
4 9 9 7 0 3 3 6 8 9 4 1 2 4
3 4 4 6 0 5 3 6 1 8 8 9 8 6

053618	309299	623904
156271	453321	633079
185173	479068	788167
191206	490451	928088
259545	544124	939109
283391	555886	984428

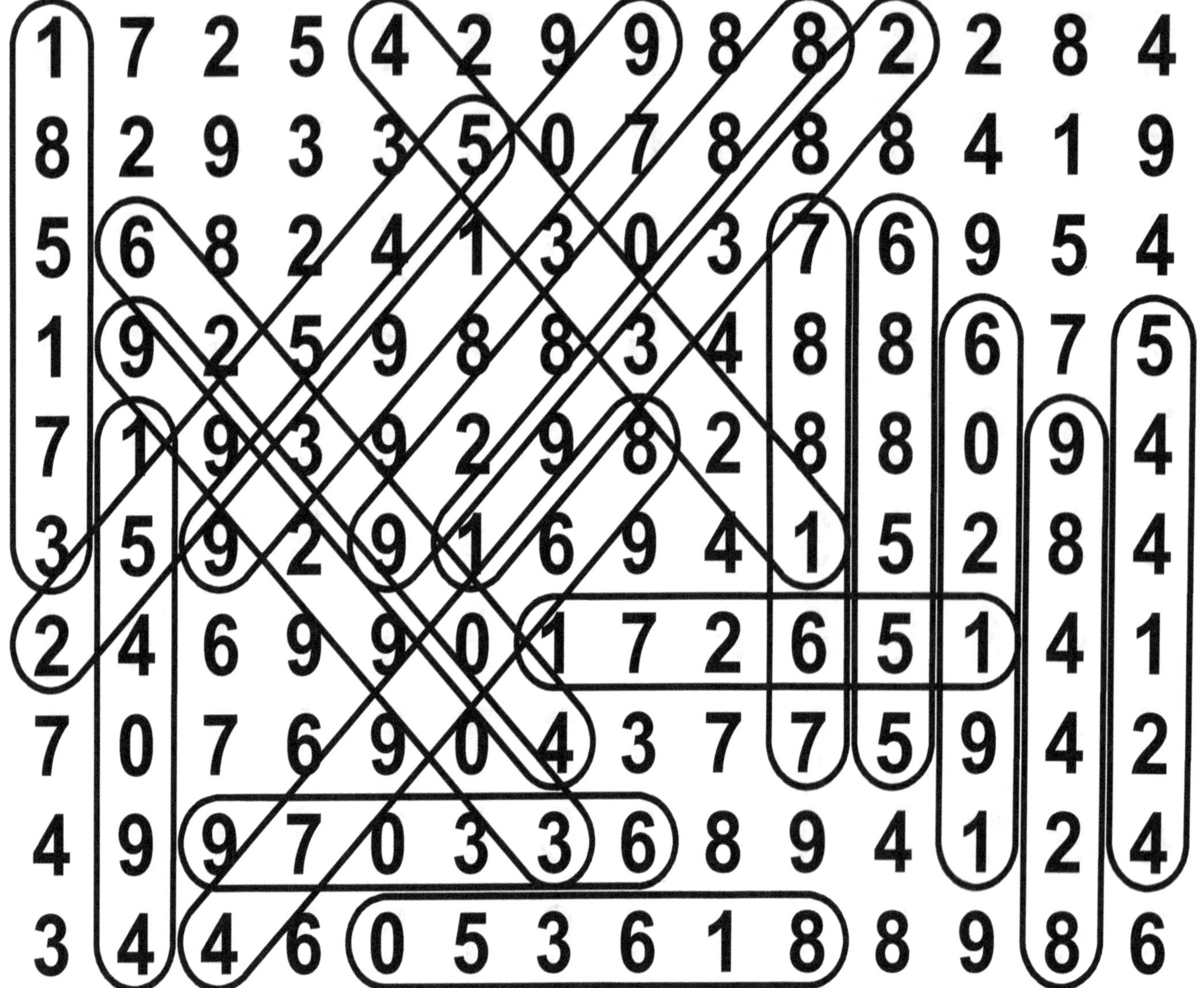

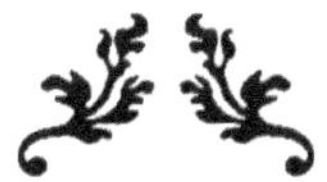

Sudoku Puzzle Section

Enjoy the following Sudoku Puzzles, ranging in difficulty from Very Easy to Hard.

Find instructions on the next page.

HOW TO SOLVE SUDOKU

Fill the 9×9 grid with digits so that <u>each column</u>, <u>each row</u>, and <u>each of the nine 3×3 sub-grids</u> that compose the grid contains digits from 1 to 9.

5	3	4	6	7	8	9	1	2
6	7	2	1	9	5	3	4	8
1	9	8	3	4	2	5	6	7
8	5	9	7	6	1	4	2	3
4	2	6	8	5	3	7	9	1
7	1	3	9	2	4	8	5	6
9	6	1	5	3	7	2	8	4
2	8	7	4	1	9	6	3	5
3	4	5	2	8	6	1	7	9

The same single number *may not appear twice* in the same row, column, or sub-grids.

SUDOKU PUZZLE #1 – VERY EASY

Each column, each row, & each of the nine 3×3 sub-grids contain all digits 1 to 9 without duplicating any digits!

PUZZLE #1 SOLUTION

1	6	5	3	2	7	9	8	4
3	8	7	5	9	4	6	2	1
4	9	2	1	6	8	3	7	5
7	3	4	2	5	6	8	1	9
9	1	6	8	4	3	7	5	2
2	5	8	7	1	9	4	6	3
5	4	3	6	8	1	2	9	7
8	2	9	4	7	5	1	3	6
6	7	1	9	3	2	5	4	8

SUDOKU PUZZLE #2 – VERY EASY

Each column, each row, & each of the nine 3×3 sub-grids contains all digits 1 to 9 without duplicating any digits!

PUZZLE #2 SOLUTION

1	2	8	3	6	5	9	7	4
3	5	4	9	7	8	6	1	2
6	7	9	4	1	2	8	5	3
2	3	5	8	9	7	4	6	1
8	4	1	6	5	3	2	9	7
9	6	7	2	4	1	5	3	8
4	9	2	7	3	6	1	8	5
5	8	3	1	2	9	7	4	6
7	1	6	5	8	4	3	2	9

SUDOKU PUZZLE #3 – VERY EASY

Each column, each row, & each of the nine 3×3 sub-grids contains all digits 1 to 9 without duplicating any digits!

PUZZLE #3 SOLUTION

8	2	6	5	9	4	1	7	3
7	5	9	6	1	3	4	8	2
4	3	1	8	2	7	6	5	9
5	1	8	4	3	9	7	2	6
3	4	7	2	5	6	8	9	1
6	9	2	7	8	1	3	4	5
9	6	4	1	7	2	5	3	8
1	8	3	9	4	5	2	6	7
2	7	5	3	6	8	9	1	4

SUDOKU PUZZLE #4 – EASY

			4	3		1	6	
			1					
			8	5		9		
1						4		7
	5							
	8	2	6		1	5		
			9					4
		5				7		
3	2		5				8	

Each column, each row, & each of the nine 3×3 sub-grids contains all digits 1 to 9 without duplicating any digits!

PUZZLE #4 SOLUTION

2	7	8	4	3	9	1	6	5
5	9	4	1	2	6	3	7	8
6	3	1	8	5	7	9	4	2
1	6	9	3	8	5	4	2	7
4	5	3	7	9	2	8	1	6
7	8	2	6	4	1	5	9	3
8	1	6	9	7	3	2	5	4
9	4	5	2	6	8	7	3	1
3	2	7	5	1	4	6	8	9

SUDOKU PUZZLE #5 – EASY

Each column, each row, & each of the nine 3×3 sub-grids contains all digits 1 to 9 without duplicating any digits!

PUZZLE #5 SOLUTION

5	6	2	7	4	1	9	8	3
8	1	4	3	2	9	7	6	5
7	9	3	5	8	6	1	2	4
2	5	6	4	1	7	8	3	9
1	7	9	8	3	5	2	4	6
4	3	8	9	6	2	5	1	7
9	4	1	6	5	8	3	7	2
6	8	5	2	7	3	4	9	1
3	2	7	1	9	4	6	5	8

SUDOKU PUZZLE #6 – EASY

Each column, each row, & each of the
nine 3×3 sub-grids contains all digits
1 to 9 without duplicating any digits!

PUZZLE #6 SOLUTION

3	2	8	7	6	9	1	5	4
1	7	5	4	3	2	6	9	8
4	9	6	1	5	8	7	3	2
9	4	1	5	8	7	3	2	6
8	5	2	6	4	3	9	1	7
7	6	3	2	9	1	4	8	5
5	1	7	3	2	4	8	6	9
6	3	9	8	7	5	2	4	1
2	8	4	9	1	6	5	7	3

SUDOKU PUZZLE #7 – MEDIUM

Each column, each row, & each of the nine 3×3 sub-grids contains all digits 1 to 9 without duplicating any digits!

PUZZLE #7 SOLUTION

4	6	9	7	1	2	5	8	3
7	1	2	8	3	5	9	4	6
5	8	3	4	6	9	2	7	1
9	7	1	5	2	6	8	3	4
2	5	8	3	4	7	1	6	9
6	3	4	1	9	8	7	2	5
8	4	7	9	5	3	6	1	2
1	2	5	6	7	4	3	9	8
3	9	6	2	8	1	4	5	7

SUDOKU PUZZLE #8 – MEDIUM

9	5				3			7
		4	5			1		9
	2							
		7		1				
				5				1
	4	6	2					
4	7	8			2			
			3	4			9	
		2					6	

Each column, each row, & each of the nine 3×3 sub-grids contains all digits 1 to 9 without duplicating any digits!

PUZZLE #8 SOLUTION

9	5	1	4	6	3	2	8	7
8	6	4	5	2	7	1	3	9
7	2	3	9	8	1	6	5	4
5	3	7	8	1	4	9	2	6
2	8	9	7	5	6	3	4	1
1	4	6	2	3	9	8	7	5
4	7	8	6	9	2	5	1	3
6	1	5	3	4	8	7	9	2
3	9	2	1	7	5	4	6	8

SUDOKU PUZZLE #9 – MEDIUM

Each column, each row, & each of the nine 3×3 sub-grids contains all digits 1 to 9 without duplicating any digits!

PUZZLE #9 SOLUTION

5	6	2	7	3	9	4	8	1
7	8	4	2	1	5	3	9	6
3	1	9	6	8	4	5	2	7
6	7	1	9	4	3	8	5	2
4	3	5	8	7	2	1	6	9
2	9	8	5	6	1	7	3	4
8	4	7	3	9	6	2	1	5
1	2	6	4	5	8	9	7	3
9	5	3	1	2	7	6	4	8

SUDOKU PUZZLE #10 – HARD

Each column, each row, & each of the nine 3×3 sub-grids contains all digits 1 to 9 without duplicating any digits!

PUZZLE #10 SOLUTION

6	8	7	1	3	4	2	5	9
5	3	9	2	8	7	6	4	1
1	2	4	5	9	6	8	3	7
3	7	8	6	4	2	9	1	5
4	1	6	9	5	8	3	7	2
2	9	5	7	1	3	4	8	6
9	6	3	8	7	5	1	2	4
8	5	1	4	2	9	7	6	3
7	4	2	3	6	1	5	9	8

SUDOKU PUZZLE #11 – HARD

Each column, each row, & each of the nine 3×3 sub-grids contains all digits 1 to 9 without duplicating any digits!

PUZZLE #11 SOLUTION

3	9	4	2	8	5	7	1	6
6	5	2	9	1	7	3	8	4
7	1	8	4	6	3	5	2	9
1	4	7	5	2	6	8	9	3
2	6	3	7	9	8	1	4	5
5	8	9	3	4	1	2	6	7
8	7	6	1	3	9	4	5	2
9	2	5	8	7	4	6	3	1
4	3	1	6	5	2	9	7	8

SUDOKU PUZZLE #12 – HARD

Each column, each row, & each of the nine 3×3 sub-grids contains all digits 1 to 9 without duplicating any digits!

PUZZLE #12 SOLUTION

9	7	6	1	2	8	5	3	4
8	3	1	4	9	5	6	7	2
5	2	4	7	3	6	9	8	1
7	4	9	8	6	1	3	2	5
2	6	5	3	4	9	7	1	8
3	1	8	5	7	2	4	9	6
4	9	2	6	1	7	8	5	3
6	5	7	2	8	3	1	4	9
1	8	3	9	5	4	2	6	7

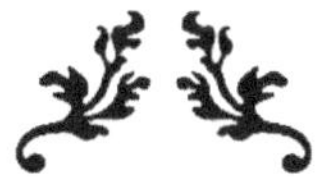

Wordoku Puzzle Section

Wordoku puzzles are solved just like Sudoku puzzles using each letter in the given word once in each grid, column and row.

Find instructions on the next page.

HOW TO SOLVE WORDOKU

Fill the 9×9 grid with the letters of the word given so that each column, each row, and each of the nine 3×3 sub-grids contains all the letters in the word. The same single letter _may not appear_ _twice_ in the same row, column, or sub-grid.

D	S	I	C	Y	O	V	E	R
R	C	V	E	I	D	S	O	Y
O	Y	E	S	R	V	I	D	C
I	D	Y	R	O	C	E	S	V
C	R	O	V	S	E	D	Y	I
E	V	S	Y	D	I	C	R	O
V	E	R	D	C	Y	O	I	S
S	O	C	I	E	R	Y	V	D
Y	I	D	O	V	S	R	C	E

DISCOVERY

WORDOKU #1

WORD TO USE: ADJUSTING

Each column, each row, & each of the nine 3×3 sub-grids contains all letters of the word without any duplicates!

WORDOKU #1 SOLUTION

S	G	J	I	U	D	A	N	T
I	U	T	A	N	S	G	D	J
A	D	N	J	T	G	S	U	I
G	T	A	N	I	U	J	S	D
D	N	S	T	G	J	U	I	A
J	I	U	S	D	A	N	T	G
T	S	G	D	J	N	I	A	U
U	A	I	G	S	T	D	J	N
N	J	D	U	A	I	T	G	S

WORDOKU #2

C		A						W
		K				E		
		T						
R							C	
	T	E	S					K
		S		T	U			A
K		W	U					C
				A				
			W	K			U	T

WORD TO USE: AWESTRUCK

Each column, each row, & each of the nine 3×3 sub-grids contains all letters of the word without any duplicates!

WORDOKU #2 SOLUTION

C	R	A	T	U	E	K	S	W
U	S	K	A	C	W	E	T	R
E	W	T	R	S	K	C	A	U
R	K	U	E	W	A	T	C	S
A	T	E	S	R	C	U	W	K
W	C	S	K	T	U	R	E	A
K	A	W	U	E	T	S	R	C
T	U	R	C	A	S	W	K	E
S	E	C	W	K	R	A	U	T

WORDOKU #3

WORD TO USE: BACKSLIDE

Each column, each row, & each of the nine 3×3 sub-grids contains all letters of the word without any duplicates!

WORDOKU #3 SOLUTION

B	E	D	I	K	A	S	C	L
C	A	I	L	E	S	D	K	B
L	S	K	B	C	D	I	E	A
I	D	L	E	S	B	K	A	C
A	C	B	K	D	I	E	L	S
E	K	S	A	L	C	B	I	D
D	I	A	C	B	E	L	S	K
K	B	C	S	I	L	A	D	E
S	L	E	D	A	K	C	B	I

WORDOKU #4

WORD TO USE: BIRTHDAYS

Each column, each row, & each of the nine 3×3 sub-grids contains all letters of the word without any duplicates!

WORDOKU #4 SOLUTION

A	D	I	R	T	S	H	B	Y
R	H	S	B	D	Y	A	I	T
Y	T	B	H	I	A	D	R	S
I	B	D	A	Y	R	T	S	H
T	S	Y	I	H	D	B	A	R
H	R	A	S	B	T	Y	D	I
S	A	H	Y	R	B	I	T	D
B	Y	T	D	S	I	R	H	A
D	I	R	T	A	H	S	Y	B

WORDOKU #5

WORD TO USE: CHEMISTRY

Each column, each row, & each of the nine 3×3 sub-grids contains all letters of the word without any duplicates!

WORDOKU #5 SOLUTION

S	E	H	T	M	C	Y	I	R
I	T	M	E	Y	R	S	C	H
Y	C	R	H	S	I	M	T	E
M	R	S	I	C	T	H	E	Y
E	I	C	R	H	Y	T	S	M
T	H	Y	S	E	M	I	R	C
R	Y	T	M	I	E	C	H	S
H	M	I	C	R	S	E	Y	T
C	S	E	Y	T	H	R	M	I

WORDOKU #6

WORD TO USE: CONSULATE

Each column, each row, & each of the nine 3×3 sub-grids contains all letters of the word without any duplicates!

WORDOKU #6 SOLUTION

L	U	N	C	O	S	A	T	E
A	C	S	T	N	E	L	U	O
O	E	T	U	L	A	N	S	C
T	A	L	N	E	U	O	C	S
N	O	U	A	S	C	T	E	L
E	S	C	O	T	L	U	A	N
C	L	A	E	U	N	S	O	T
S	T	E	L	A	O	C	N	U
U	N	O	S	C	T	E	L	A

WORDOKU #7

WORD TO USE: DISCOVERY

Each column, each row, & each of the nine 3×3 sub-grids contains all letters of the word without any duplicates!

WORDOKU #7 SOLUTION

D	S	I	C	Y	O	V	E	R
R	C	V	E	I	D	S	O	Y
O	Y	E	S	R	V	I	D	C
I	D	Y	R	O	C	E	S	V
C	R	O	V	S	E	D	Y	I
E	V	S	Y	D	I	C	R	O
V	E	R	D	C	Y	O	I	S
S	O	C	I	E	R	Y	V	D
Y	I	D	O	V	S	R	C	E

WORDOKU #8

WORD TO USE: EDUCATION

Each column, each row, & each of the nine 3×3 sub-grids contains all letters of the word without any duplicates!

WORDOKU #8 SOLUTION

O	E	T	N	A	D	C	U	I
I	U	A	E	O	C	D	T	N
D	C	N	T	I	U	A	O	E
T	I	D	O	N	A	E	C	U
E	A	U	C	D	T	I	N	O
C	N	O	I	U	E	T	A	D
U	D	I	A	T	N	O	E	C
A	O	E	U	C	I	N	D	T
N	T	C	D	E	O	U	I	A

WORDOKU #9

WORD TO USE: FLOWERING

Each column, each row, & each of the nine 3×3 sub-grids contains all letters of the word without any duplicates!

WORDOKU #9 SOLUTION

N	I	O	R	F	W	G	L	E
L	E	F	N	G	O	I	R	W
G	W	R	L	E	I	O	N	F
W	N	I	E	O	L	F	G	R
R	O	E	F	W	G	L	I	N
F	G	L	I	R	N	E	W	O
O	F	G	W	L	R	N	E	I
I	L	W	O	N	E	R	F	G
E	R	N	G	I	F	W	O	L

WORDOKU #10

WORD TO USE: HARMONIZE

Each column, each row, & each of the nine 3×3 sub-grids contains all letters of the word without any duplicates!

WORDOKU #10 SOLUTION

A	N	M	H	E	I	Z	R	O
R	I	H	Z	N	O	E	A	M
O	Z	E	R	A	M	I	H	N
M	R	N	I	H	Z	A	O	E
E	O	I	N	M	A	H	Z	R
H	A	Z	E	O	R	N	M	I
N	H	O	A	R	E	M	I	Z
Z	M	A	O	I	N	R	E	H
I	E	R	M	Z	H	O	N	A

WORDOKU #11

	L							
				U		C	I	E
		E		T	R			
	A		I					
T		C				A		
							C	
	T		A					
V						U		T
E		U		C	L			

WORD TO USE: LUCRATIVE

Each column, each row, & each of the nine 3×3 sub-grids contains all letters of the word without any duplicates!

WORDOKU #11 SOLUTION

C	L	V	E	I	A	T	U	R
A	R	T	L	U	V	C	I	E
I	U	E	C	T	R	V	A	L
U	A	L	I	R	C	E	T	V
T	V	C	U	L	E	A	R	I
R	E	I	V	A	T	L	C	U
L	T	R	A	V	U	I	E	C
V	C	A	R	E	I	U	L	T
E	I	U	T	C	L	R	V	A

WORDOKU #12

WORD TO USE: SYMPHONIC

Each column, each row, & each of the nine 3×3 sub-grids contains all letters of the word without any duplicates!

WORDOKU #12 SOLUTION

O	M	H	C	Y	N	S	I	P
I	P	C	S	O	H	N	Y	M
N	S	Y	P	I	M	C	O	H
P	Y	S	I	H	C	O	M	N
C	N	I	O	M	Y	P	H	S
H	O	M	N	P	S	I	C	Y
M	C	O	Y	N	P	H	S	I
S	H	P	M	C	I	Y	N	O
Y	I	N	H	S	O	M	P	C

"May the LORD bless you and protect you. May the LORD smile on you and be gracious to you. May the LORD show you his favor and give you his peace."

~ Numbers 6:24-26

Thank you for your purchase! If you enjoyed solving these puzzles, would you help us help others by giving us a positive review on Amazon?

Find all the Supersized Puzzle books at **amazon.com/author/ninaporter**! Or just search for:
Supersized for Challenged Eyes

Check out **SupersizedPuzzles.com**
Sign up to receive FREE printable:
- ✓ Weekly Puzzles
- ✓ Puzzle 4-Pack Download

Find us on **Facebook**
@supersizedpuzzles

www.ingramcontent.com/pod-product-compliance
Lightning Source LLC
Chambersburg PA
CBHW080304030726
47593CB00009B/2622